# RESPIRATORY THERAPY PHARMACOLOGY

## JOSEPH L. RAU, JR., M.A., R.R.T.

*Department of Respiratory Therapy*
*College of Allied Health Sciences*
*Georgia State University*

## YEAR BOOK MEDICAL PUBLISHERS, INC.

Chicago • London

*Reprinted, March 1979*

Library of Congress Catalog Card Number: 77-90061

International Standard Book Number: 0-8151-7075-0

# Preface

RESPIRATORY THERAPY PHARMACOLOGY represents one area of drug application, which can be summarized as the area of bronchoactive drugs. Respiratory therapy pharmacology is even more specific than general pharmacology, which is itself an applied field of study resting on more fundamental sciences such as chemistry and biology. Generally, the specific drugs utilized in respiratory care are delivered by aerosol, another distinguishing characteristic. The group of bronchoactive drugs is intended to provide pharmacologic care of the airway, either through control of bronchial smooth muscle, or through control of secretions. Seven categories of drugs used directly by respiratory therapy are currently included in the bronchoactive group, offering a diversely challenging field of study. In each category of drugs considered in the text, a brief review of the underlying pharmacology and physiology is first offered, and then specific drugs are identified for review. A general introductory consideration of basic pharmacologic principles and the autonomic nervous system is included, as well as drug dosage calculations, with practice problems and answers. Several drug categories (neuromuscular blockers, prostaglandins) not directly used by respiratory therapists are also discussed.

The material considered ranges from the factual and simple to the theoretical and complex, in the hope of providing useful information for all levels of personnel engaged in respiratory care. Limitation of scope to respiratory therapy drugs and drugs directly related to respiratory care is deliberate, in the belief that the field has evolved to the point of requiring in-depth treatment of well-defined subjects, rather than a comprehensive review of all topics within one text.

# Acknowledgments

The writing of any text demands as much sacrifice from the writer's family, as from the writer. My wife, Mary, and son, Joseph, have both provided the cooperation and encouragement needed to complete the task. The efforts of good friends and past teachers, William Grosse, Ph.D., and John Holbrook, Ph.D., are deeply appreciated. The greatest indebtedness however is to the students in R.T. 245 (pharmacology), current and past, whose inquiring minds and need for knowledge have constantly inspired a continuing effort to organize the material presented. Sincere and grateful appreciation is extended to the following members of the Educational Media Department at Georgia State University, who expertly provided all of the artwork: Phyllis Brown, Ruthanne Mitchell, Leita Cowart, William Biggers, and Paul Brown. Ms. Mo Brooks has patiently coordinated typing, arranging, and proofing of the text with admirable care.

*"If I have seen further, it is by standing on the shoulders of giants."*
Isaac Newton, letter to Robert Hooke, February 5, 1675

JOSEPH L. RAU, JR.

# Table of Contents

1. **General Principles of Pharmacology** . . . . . . . . . . 1
   Definition of Terms. . . . . . . . . . . . . . 1
   Legislation Affecting Drugs. . . . . . . . . . . . 2
   Naming Drugs . . . . . . . . . . . . . . 2
   Sources of Drugs . . . . . . . . . . . . . 3
   Sources of Drug Information . . . . . . . . . . 3
   Receptor Theory of Drug Action . . . . . . . . . . 4
   Basic Drug Concepts . . . . . . . . . . . . 6
   Drug Interactions . . . . . . . . . . . . . 8
   Drug Absorption. . . . . . . . . . . . . . 9
      Passive Transfer. . . . . . . . . . . . . . 10
      Specialized Transport. . . . . . . . . . . . . 11
   Dosage Forms and Routes of Administration . . . . . . . 11
      Oral Route. . . . . . . . . . . . . . . 12
      Parenteral Route . . . . . . . . . . . . . 12
      Inhalation Route . . . . . . . . . . . . . 13
      Topical Route—Mucous Membranes . . . . . . . . 16
      Topical Route—Skin Application . . . . . . . . . 16
   The Prescription . . . . . . . . . . . . . . 17
   Medication Teaching Card. . . . . . . . . . . . 20
   Respiratory Therapy Pharmacology—A Comprehensive
      Overview. . . . . . . . . . . . . . . . . 20

2. **Calculating Drug Dosages**. . . . . . . . . . . . 23
   The Metric System . . . . . . . . . . . . . . 23
   The Apothecary System. . . . . . . . . . . . . 24
   The Avoirdupois System . . . . . . . . . . . . 25
   Intersystem Conversions . . . . . . . . . . . . 26
      Approximate Equivalents . . . . . . . . . . . 26
   Drug Dosage Calculation . . . . . . . . . . . . 27
   Calculating Dosages from Prepared-Strength Liquids,
      Tablets, and Capsules . . . . . . . . . . . . 27

Calculating Dosages from Percentage-Strength Solutions. . . . . 29
   Types of Percentage Preparations . . . . . . . . . . . . 30
   Solving Percentage and Solution Problems . . . . . . . . 31
Solutions: Definitions and Terms . . . . . . . . . . . . 33

**3. The Central and Peripheral Nervous System** . . . . . . . . **35**
Autonomic Nervous System . . . . . . . . . . . . 37
   Parasympathetic Branch. . . . . . . . . . . . 37
Sympathetic Branch . . . . . . . . . . . . . . 39
Terminology of Drugs Affecting the Autonomic Nervous System . . 43
Unified Theory of Autonomic Control in Lung . . . . . . . 44

**4. Sympathomimetic Bronchodilators**. . . . . . . . . . . . . **49**
Specific Sympathomimetic Bronchodilators. . . . . . . . . . 51
   Epinephrine HCl . . . . . . . . . . . . . . 51
   Racemic epinephrine (Micronefrin, Vaponefrin) . . . . . . 53
   Isoproterenol (Isuprel) . . . . . . . . . . . 54
   Isoproterenol and cyclopentamine (Aerolone) . . . . . . 56
   Isoetharine and phenylephrine (Bronkosol) . . . . . . . 56
   Metaproterenol sulfate (Alupent, Metaprel, or ciprenaline) . . . 57
   Terbutaline sulfate (Bricanyl, Brethine) . . . . . . . 57
   Salbutamol (albuterol) . . . . . . . . . . . 58
Problems with Mistometer Delivery Systems . . . . . . . . 59

**5. Parasympatholytic and Xanthine Bronchodilators** . . . . . . . **61**
Parasympatholytic Agents . . . . . . . . . . . . 62
   Atropine sulfate. . . . . . . . . . . . . . 63
   Aerosol Sch 1000 (ipratropium bromide) . . . . . . . . 63
Xanthine Agents . . . . . . . . . . . . . . 64
   Theophylline ethylenediamine (aminophylline) . . . . . 65
   Theophylline capsules (Elixophyllin) . . . . . . . . 65
   Theophylline elixir (Elixophyllin) . . . . . . . . . 66
   Ephedrine, theophylline, glyceryl guaiacolate, and
     phenobarbital (Bronkotabs) . . . . . . . . . . 66
   Theophylline and guaifenesin (Asbron G) . . . . . . 66

**6. Mucolytics** . . . . . . . . . . . . . . **68**
Physiology and Nature of Mucus . . . . . . . . . . . 68

Specific Mucolytic Agents . . . . . . . . . . . . . 70

    Humidifiers . . . . . . . . . . . . . . . . 70

    Acetylcysteine (Mucomyst, Mucomyst-10) . . . . . . . . 71

    Pancreatic dornase (Dornavac) . . . . . . . . . . . 73

    Sodium bicarbonate . . . . . . . . . . . . . . 73

    Clinical Use of Mucolytics . . . . . . . . . . . . 74

**7. Surface-active Agents** . . . . . . . . . . . . . . **77**

    Specific Surface-active Agents . . . . . . . . . . . 79

    Alcohol (ethanol, ethyl alcohol) . . . . . . . . . . 79

    Tyloxapol (Alevaire) . . . . . . . . . . . . . 80

    Sodium ethasulfate (Tergemist) . . . . . . . . . . 81

    Clinical Consideration of Surface-active Agents . . . . . . 81

**8. Corticosteroids in Respiratory Therapy** . . . . . . . . . **83**

    Anatomy and Physiology of Corticosteroids . . . . . . . 84

    Structure-Activity Relations of Corticosteroids . . . . . . 85

    Neurosecretory Control of Adrenal Cortex . . . . . . . 87

    Pharmacology and Effects of Glucocorticoids . . . . . . . 89

    Anti-inflammatory Effects . . . . . . . . . . . . 89

    Enhanced Bronchodilation . . . . . . . . . . . . 90

    Immunosuppression . . . . . . . . . . . . . 90

    General Physiologic Effects . . . . . . . . . . . 91

    Diurnal Rhythms and Alternate-Day Therapy . . . . . . 91

    Aerosol vs Oral Therapy . . . . . . . . . . . . 92

    Specific Aerosol Corticosteroids . . . . . . . . . . 93

    Dexamethasone sodium phosphate (Decadron) . . . . . . 93

    Beclomethasone dipropionate (Vanceril) . . . . . . . . 94

    Triamcinolone acetonide . . . . . . . . . . . . 94

**9. Cromolyn Sodium: Antiasthmatic** . . . . . . . . . . . **96**

    Physiology of Allergic Asthma . . . . . . . . . . . 96

    Cromolyn sodium (Intal, Aarane) . . . . . . . . . . 100

**10. Antibiotics in Respiratory Therapy** . . . . . . . . . . **104**

    Modes of Action . . . . . . . . . . . . . . 104

    Clinical Aspects of Antibiotics . . . . . . . . . . . 105

    Aerosolized Antibiotics in Respiratory Care . . . . . . . 107

11. **Skeletal Muscle Relaxants (Neuromuscular Blocking Agents)** . . **110**

    Physiology of the Myoneural Junction . . . . . . . . . . . 111

    Neuromuscular Blockers . . . . . . . . . . . . . . . . 111

       Nondepolarizing Blockers . . . . . . . . . . . . . . . 111

       Depolarizing Blockers . . . . . . . . . . . . . . . . 113

    Nondepolarizing Neuromuscular Blocking Agents . . . . . . . 114

       *d*-Tubocurarine (tubocurarine chloride) . . . . . . . . . 114

       Dimethyl tubocurarine chloride (Mecostrin) . . . . . . . 114

       Dimethyl tubocurarine iodide (Metubine) . . . . . . . . 115

       Gallamine triethiodide (Flaxedil) . . . . . . . . . . . 115

       Pancuronium (Pavulon) . . . . . . . . . . . . . . . 115

    Depolarizing Neuromuscular Blocking Agents . . . . . . . 115

       Succinylcholine chloride (Anectine, Quelicin) . . . . . . 115

       Decamethonium (Syncurine) . . . . . . . . . . . . . 116

12. **Prostaglandins** . . . . . . . . . . . . . . . . . . **117**

    Basic Description of Prostaglandins . . . . . . . . . . . 117

       Pharmacologic Effects . . . . . . . . . . . . . . . 119

       Mode of Action . . . . . . . . . . . . . . . . . . 119

    Clinical Aspects of Prostaglandins . . . . . . . . . . . 120

13. **Systems of Drug Distribution in Respiratory Therapy** . . . . . **123**

    Separate-Syringe Method . . . . . . . . . . . . . . . 123

    Single-Syringe Method . . . . . . . . . . . . . . . . 124

    Open-Cup Method . . . . . . . . . . . . . . . . . . 124

    Unit-Dose Method . . . . . . . . . . . . . . . . . . 125

    General Suggestions for Drug Preparation in Respiratory Therapy 125

14. **Mathematics of Drug Dosage Calculation and Dosage Problems** **128**

    Arithmetic Pretest . . . . . . . . . . . . . . . . . . 128

    Arithmetic Exercises . . . . . . . . . . . . . . . . . 130

       Roman Numerals . . . . . . . . . . . . . . . . . . 131

       Fractions . . . . . . . . . . . . . . . . . . . . . 132

       Decimals . . . . . . . . . . . . . . . . . . . . . 135

       Ratios . . . . . . . . . . . . . . . . . . . . . . 136

       Percentages . . . . . . . . . . . . . . . . . . . . 137

Drug Dosage Problems . . . . . . . . . . . . . . . 139
  Conversion Calculation Problems . . . . . . . . . . . 139
  Examples of Problems on Solutions . . . . . . . . . . 140
  Problems on Solutions . . . . . . . . . . . . . . . 142
  Problems on Drug Dosage Calculation . . . . . . . . . 142

**Index** . . . . . . . . . . . . . . . . . . . . . **145**

# CHAPTER 1

# General Principles
# of Pharmacology

THE STUDY of respiratory therapy pharmacology represents a specialty area, and as such, presupposes a background of general pharmacologic principles, as well as more fundamental studies of chemistry, biology, biochemistry, anatomy, and human physiology. Certain key fundamental terms and concepts of pharmacology are included as an introductory review to facilitate comprehension of the respiratory therapy specialty.

## DEFINITION OF TERMS

*Drugs:* The many complex functions of the human organism are regulated by chemical agents such as hormones, kinins, and catecholamines. Chemicals interact with the organism to alter its function, thus illuminating the life processes, and at times providing methods of diagnosis, treatment, or prevention of disease. Such chemicals are called drugs. Most simply and universally, a drug is any chemical which alters the organism's functions or processes. Examples include oxygen, alcohol, LSD, and vitamins.

*Pharmacology:* The study of the interactions of drugs (chemicals) with the organism. This is the most general statement of the field, and includes more particular, specialized aspects, such as the drug effect within the living system (pharmacodynamics), the preparation and dispensation (pharmacy), the harmful effects of drugs (toxicology), the art of treating disease with drugs (therapeutics), that group of drugs able to destroy invading organisms without destroying the host (chemotherapy), and the sources of drugs (pharmacognosy).

## LEGISLATION AFFECTING DRUGS

1906—The first Food and Drugs Act passed by Congress. The *United States Pharmacopeia* (USP) and the *National Formulary* (NF) were given official status.

1914—The Harrison Narcotic Act to control the importation, sale, and distribution of opium and its derivatives, as well as other narcotic analgesics.

1938—The Food, Drug and Cosmetic Act became law. This is the current Federal Food, Drug and Cosmetic Act to protect the public health, and protect physicians from irresponsible drug manufacturers. This act is enforced by the Food and Drug Administration (FDA) of the Department of Health, Education, and Welfare.

1952—The Durham-Humphrey Amendment defines the drugs that may be sold by the pharmacist only on prescription.

1962—The Kefauver-Harris Act passed as an amendment to the Food, Drug and Cosmetic Act of 1938. This act requires proof of safety and efficacy of all drugs introduced since 1938. Drugs in use prior to that time have not been reviewed but are under study.

May 1, 1971—The Controlled Substances Act became effective; this act lists requirements for the control, sale, and dispensation of narcotics and dangerous drugs. Five schedules of controlled substances have been defined. Schedule I to schedule V generally define drugs of decreasing potential for abuse, increasing medical use, and decreasing physical dependence. Examples of each schedule follow:

Schedule I—heroin, marijuana, LSD, peyote, and mescaline.

Schedule II—opium, morphine, codeine, cocaine, amphetamines.

Schedule III—glutethimide (Doriden), paregoric, and barbiturates, with some exceptions.

Schedule IV—phenobarbital, barbital, chloral hydrate, meprobamate (Equanil, Miltown), and paraldehyde.

Schedule V—narcotics containing non-narcotics in mixture form, such as cough preparations or Lomotil.

## NAMING DRUGS

*Chemical name:* This is the drug's structural formula.

*Official name:* This name, which may be identical with the generic name, is issued by the USP or the NF.

*Generic name:* This is the name assigned by the laboratory or company developing the drug, and may be an abbreviated form of the chemical name.

*Trade name:* This is the brand or trade name of the drug given by a particular manufacturer or seller of the drug.

For example, Beclomethasone

Chemical name: 9α-chloro-11β,17α,21-trihydroxy-16β-methylpregna-1,4-diene-3,20-dione 17,21-dipropionate

Official name: beclomethasone dipropionate

Generic name: beclomethasone dipropionate

Trade name: Vanceril

## SOURCES OF DRUGS

Although the sources of drugs is not a crucial area of expertise for the respiratory care clinician, it can be one of the most interesting. Recognition of naturally occurring drugs dates back to Egyptian papyrus records, to the ancient Chinese, to the Central American civilizations, and is still seen in remote regions of the United States such as Appalachia.

The prototype of cromolyn sodium was khellin, found in the Eastern Mediterranean plant *Ammi visnaga,* and the plant was used in ancient times as a muscle relaxant. Today its synthetic derivative is used as an antiasthmatic agent. Similar stories can be traced for curare, derived from large vines and used by South American Indians to coat their arrow tips for lethal effect; for digitalis, obtained from the foxglove plant *(Digitalis purpurea),* reputedly used by the Mayans for relief of angina, and definitely referred to by thirteenth-century Welsh physicians; and of course for the notorious poppy seed, source of the opium alkaloids, immortalized in *Confessions of an English Opium Eater.*

Today, the most common source of drugs is chemical synthesis, but plants, minerals, and animals have often contributed the prototype of the active ingredient. Examples of each source can be given:

Animal—thyroid hormone, insulin, pancreatic dornase.

Plant—khellin *(Ammi visnaga),* atropine *(belladonna* alkaloid), digitalis (foxglove), reserpine *(Rauwolfia serpentina),* volatile oils of eucalyptus, pine, anise.

Mineral—copper sulfate, magnesium sulfate (Epsom salts), mineral oil (liquid hydrocarbons).

## SOURCES OF DRUG INFORMATION

The two official volumes giving drug standards in the United States are:

*The United States Pharmacopeia* (USP)—first published in 1820 as a private medical effort; given official status in 1906 with the first congressional Food and Drugs Act. The *Pharmacopeia* specifies standards for such drugs as oxygen, indicated by the USP label. The *Pharmacopeia* undergoes revision every five years.

*The National Formulary* (NF)—first published in 1888, and has the same legal status as the USP. It is published by the American Pharmaceutical Association, and is revised continuously.

Other sources of drug information are:

*AMA Drug Evaluations*—gives information and results on new drugs which are not yet officially included in the USP.

*Physicians' Desk Reference* (PDR)—prepared by manufacturers of drugs, and therefore potentially lacking the objectivity of the preceding sources. This annual volume does provide useful information, including ·descriptive color charts for drug identification, names of manufacturers, and general drug actions.

*Hospital Formulary*—published by the American Society of Hospital Pharmacists, and very informative. This publication contains monographs and commentaries on classes of drugs (antibiotics, steroids, etc.).

In-depth discussion of pharmacologic principles and modes of drug action can be found in *Krantz and Carr's Pharmacologic Principles of Medical Practice* (edited by D. M. Aviado) and *The Pharmacological Basis of Therapeutics* (by L. S. Goodman, and A. Gilman).

## RECEPTOR THEORY OF DRUG ACTION

Beginning in 1878 with Langley, it has been theorized that a drug exerts its effect at a specific site in the body, and is physically in contact with that site to bring about the effect. Using a lock-and-key analogy, the site is the receptor or "lock" for which the drug is a specific key (Fig 1–1). The structure of the drug is related to the correlative structure of the receptor, and just as one key can fit one lock but not others, so one drug is specific to certain types of receptors but not others.

The essential concepts for explaining drug action are:

1.   The drug has to actually reach the receptor;

2.   A drug is specific to its matching receptor;

3.   This specificity is based on the chemical structure of the drug. The third concept is usually termed the *structure-activity relationship* of the drug, or SAR.

The receptor model explains why one drug can affect certain organs or systems but not others, why small changes in chemical structure

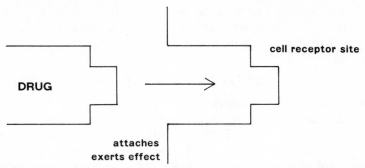

Fig 1–1.—Diagrammatic representation of drug-receptor interaction.

bring about significant changes in drug action, and how a drug can compete with endogenous chemicals to block the usual effect of those chemicals. This concept has been fruitful for developing drugs such as metaproterenol which will have an effect primarily in the lungs, instead of stimulating the beta receptors in both heart and lungs equally in the manner of isoproterenol. The difference between these two drugs is a minor change in structure. On the basis of the structure-activity relationship of phenylephrine and isoproterenol, Ahlquist differentiated alpha (peripheral blood vessels) from beta (lung, heart, skeletal muscle blood supply) receptors. Phenylephrine produced effects at sites which came to be called alpha (α), and isoproterenol activated beta (β) sites. Lands, in 1967, further differentiated beta-one and beta-two sites in the same manner. The clinical usefulness of a drug is directly related to the specificity of its action. For example, acetylcholine is a poor drug for treatment because it activates far too many receptor sites. Acetylcholine is analogous to a passkey which is universal to many locks, whereas a more specific drug such as metaproterenol can fit only one.

The autoregulation of the body is based on certain chemical keys fitting matched receptor locks. By "duplicating" the endogenous chemical key with a drug, one can mimic or block the natural chemical's effect. This is the basis of therapeutics in pharmacology.

When a drug does match a certain receptor site, an effect may be produced in several ways:

1.  Drug-receptor combination may inhibit enzymes which normally cause other reactions; thus the reactions are blocked.
2.  The drug may act as a coenzyme. Epinephrine plus adenyl cyclase catalyzes the formation of adenosine 3':5'-cyclic monophosphate (cyclic AMP).
3.  The drug may alter cell membrane permeability by interacting

with carrier mechanisms. For example, digitalis is thought to increase the availability of calcium to cardiac myocardium, causing strengthened contractions.

## BASIC DRUG CONCEPTS

When one plots the relationship of the dosage of a drug to the measured effect of the drug on a logarithmic scale, a sigmoid curve is obtained as seen in Figure 1–2. This graph or sigmoid curve is referred to as a log dose-response curve. The lowest point of such a curve would be that point at which there is no effect. At a certain threshold dose a measured effect begins to be observed. The highest point on a sigmoid curve would be the point of maximal effect, and increasing dosages above this point would produce no increasing effect (see Fig 1–2). By experimentation, one can determine the dosage of the drug that would be lethal to 50% of a test population of animals. This dose which is lethal to 50% of the population is termed the *median lethal dose,* or $LD_{50}$. One can also determine the dose which is therapeutically effective for 50% of the test population, termed the *median effective dose,* or $ED_{50}$. The ratio of the $LD_{50}$ to the $ED_{50}$ is termed the therapeutic index or TI (Fig 1–3).

**Fig 1–2.**—Curve obtained by plotting the effect of a drug against increasing dosage strength on a logarithmic scale. This is termed the log dose-response curve.

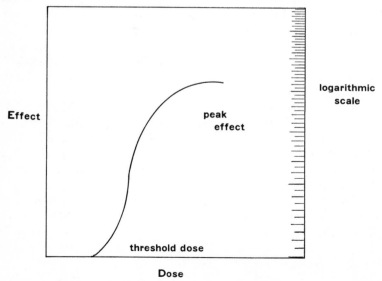

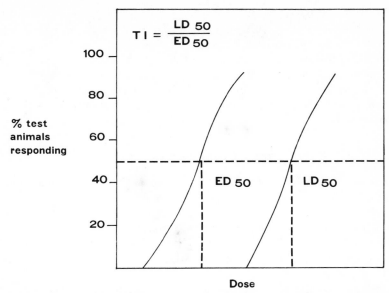

**Fig 1–3.**—Therapeutic index (*TI*) indicating the effective dose (*ED₅₀*) and the lethal dose (*LD₅₀*) for 50% of the population.

$$\text{therapeutic index} = \frac{LD_{50}}{ED_{50}}$$

In words, this index indicates how close the effective dose is to the dose which is lethal for 50% of the test population. As the $ED_{50}$ approaches the $LD_{50}$, the danger of a drug increases significantly. If the $LD_{50}$ is 9 grams, and the $ED_{50}$ is 1 gram, the TI is 9; but if the $LD_{50}$ dropped to 6 grams with an $ED_{50}$ of 4 grams, the TI would be 1.5. For example, penicillin has a therapeutic index greater than 100, which means the drug is relatively safe in terms of toxic effects or overdosage. On the other hand, digitalis has a rather low index of 1.5 to 2.0, and the toxicity or lethal level of the dose is very close to the therapeutic dose. It is interesting to note that with the increase in drug usage, the therapeutic index generally seems to decrease for all drugs.

The *potency* of a drug is based on its biologic activity per unit weight of the drug. A very potent drug has great activity for a fairly low or small unit weight. The concept of drug *efficacy* refers to the peak, or maximal effect, of the drug seen on the log dose-response curve. It is important to note that one compares drug potencies by comparing the *dosages* that produce the same effect, and not by comparing the effects produced by the same dose. The effect of a drug in a physiologic system can vary greatly because of the influence of many other variables in the system itself outside of the drug.

All of the following factors can influence the effect of a drug in the body: dose, age, body weight, sex, time of administration, rate of drug excretion, drug combinations, tolerance, and idiosyncrasy. The term *idiosyncrasy* includes all reactions to drugs not otherwise anticipated or explained.

## DRUG INTERACTIONS

With the increasing complexity of drug therapy, and because most critical patients encountered by respiratory therapy personnel are on multiple drug therapies, concepts of drug interaction become very useful for understanding patient reactions.

*Additive:* The additive effect of two drugs is basically $1 + 1 = 2$, or the two drugs together give an effect equal to the summation of their individual effects.

*Synergism:* literally translated from the Greek, means "working with." The combination of two different drugs, with one drug *inactive* on the receptor involved, produces a result greater than that of the active drug alone. This is a situation of 2 (active drug effect) + 0 (inactive drug) = 3 (total effect).

*Potentiation:* frequently used loosely in place of *synergism.* Potentiation, however, describes the effect of two drugs eliciting a response greater than the sum of each single drug's effect, or $1 + 1 = 3$. (The reader should be aware that slightly varying definitions of these terms can be found even in reference texts. Compare the texts listed at the end of this chapter.)

*Antagonism:* describes the situation of two drugs with opposing effects. For example, the effect of morphine can be reversed by use of its antagonist, nalorphine. Another example of interest to respiratory care personnel is the reversal of histamine by epinephrine.

*Cumulation:* occurs when a drug's rate of removal or inactivation is slower than the rate of administration (Fig 1–4). This can be dangerous, depending on the drug's effect, and is more likely when the drug has a long half-life in the body. The result of cumulation is toxicity, or a toxic as opposed to therapeutic level of the drug. For example, digitoxin is usually limited to 0.2 mg per day, and the ECG can be monitored for signs of toxicity (A-V block).

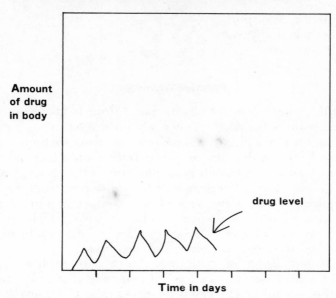

**Fig 1–4.**—Cumulative amount of a drug given daily.

*Tolerance:* the phenomenon wherein increasing amounts of a drug are needed to produce the same effect. This is variable, depending on the drug, but a well-known example is provided by the barbiturate group. Since barbiturates are metabolized in the liver by certain enzymes, this may be due to *microsomal enzyme induction,* or the increase in enzyme levels which metabolize these agents. This is due to the increasing need for the enzymes with repeated doses of barbiturates in the body.

*Tachyphylaxis:* rapidly developing tolerance, such as can occur with repeated doses of sympathomimetic compounds.

## DRUG ABSORPTION

Prior to a consideration of the routes of administration of drugs, the basic principles governing the passage of drugs across body membranes must be understood. A basic summary of these types of passage is:

1. Passive transfer
    Simple diffusion
    Filtration

2. Specialized transport
   Facilitated diffusion
   Pinocytosis

## Passive Transfer

The term *passive transfer* means that a drug is taken up across a membrane without the need for energy being exerted. Simple *diffusion* requires no energy and is the transfer of a substance across a membrane based on a difference in concentration on either side of the membrane, or a concentration gradient. This is the concept of water running downhill, and the drug will be transferred from the area of higher concentration to the area of lower concentration. The term *filtration* is used when a porous membrane exists which allows the flow of substances of a certain size only, with larger molecular sizes being blocked from passage across the membrane.

There is one factor of great importance with regard to passive transfer of a drug across a cell membrane, and that is the factor of ionization of the drug. The key principle is this: *Cell membranes are more permeable to the non-ionized form of a given drug than to an ionized form.* The basis for this is the greater lipid solubility of a non-ionized form in the cell membrane. The degree of ionization of a given drug depends on two factors: the pKa of the drug, and the ambient pH. The pKa is defined as the pH at which the drug is half ionized and half non-ionized. To put it another way, a drug is half ionized when the ambient pH equals the pKa of the drug. For example, aspirin is a weak acid whose pKa is approximately 3.5. This means that at a pH of 3.5, aspirin (acetylsalicylic acid) is 50% ionized and 50% non-ionized. The significance of this fact is that a weak acid, such as aspirin, will be less ionized in a more acidic environment, whereas a weak base, such as ephedrine or quinine, will be less ionized in a more basic environment. Thus a weak acid such as aspirin will be well absorbed from the stomach, where the pH is acidic, but quinine will not be absorbed from the stomach until it reaches the basic or less acidic intestine. The pH also influences the excretion of drugs, with the urine pH affecting the degree of diffusion of the drug.

A list of pKa values for certain weak acids and bases is given. The effect of pH on the ionization of salicylic acid (pKa = 3) and quinine, a base (pKa = 8.4), is also given to illustrate the influence of the pH on the degree of ionization.

Salicylic acid; pKa = 3  Quinine (base); pKa = 8.4
pH = 2   9% ionized    pH = 7.4  91% ionized
pH = 3  50% ionized   pH = 8.4  50% ionized
pH = 4  91% ionized   pH = 9.4   9% ionized

### Specialized Transport

Active transport of a drug refers to the situation in which the drug is moved against a concentration gradient, by the use of energy to overcome the uphill gradient.

Facilitative diffusion is a unique form of transport in which the drug attaches to a special carrier which facilitates the diffusion of the drug across the membrane and then releases the drug. The drug is not chemically altered in this process, and the carrier is free then to facilitate other drug transfer. This does require energy as in the case of active transport.

Pinocytosis describes the process of cell membranes surrounding and engulfing small droplets.

These are the basic forms of drug transfer across the cell membrane. There is a great deal of detail that is important for drug transfer with regard to the nature of the cell membrane, much of which is still theoretical and speculative, and there are other factors which influence the uptake of drugs in the body and determine which route of administration is ultimately chosen for the drug. The influence of pH in the stomach is obvious in the case of passive transfer of an ionizing drug. Another factor influencing oral versus parenteral administration of a drug would be the presence or absence of enzymes in the cell membrane to metabolize the drug. If such an enzyme were present, the drug would be metabolized (inactivated) as it was absorbed, and the chances of the drug reaching a receptor site would be considerably reduced. This is the case with isoproterenol, which is metabolized much faster during oral administration than during IV administration, or even aerosol administration. In addition to the enzyme COMT, the stomach lining possesses a second sulfatase enzyme which also inactivates isoproterenol. Thus the effect of isoproterenol when taken orally is significantly less than when taken by aerosol.

## DOSAGE FORMS AND ROUTES OF ADMINISTRATION

*Dosage form of a drug:* the product or unit in which the patient receives the drug; e.g., tablet, capsule, injection or ointment.

The route of administration depends on the following factors:
1. Whether systemic or only local effect is needed;
2. The desired rate of onset and duration of action of the drug;
3. The stability of the drug in gastric and/or intestinal fluids;
4. Whether or not the patient is able to swallow, retain, and absorb drugs given orally;
5. Convenience versus safety of various routes;
6. The amount of the drug: large amounts can be oral or IV; smaller IM, SC.

## Oral Route

The oral route is generally the safest, most convenient, and economical route for drugs intended to have systemic effect.

Dosage forms for the oral route include:
1. Tablets—solid dosage forms prepared by molding or compressing the drug in dies.
2. Capsules—contain medication within a soluble shell of gelatin, methylcellulose, or calcium alginate.
3. Pills—globular or ovoid dosage forms prepared from a cohesive, plastic mass.
4. Powders—mixtures of dry, powdered drugs. (Also used externally, e.g., dusting powders, powders for douche solutions, etc.)
5. Solutions—homogeneous mixture of a solvent and a solute. A common solvent is water.
6. Elixirs—sweetened, hydroalcoholic solutions, usually flavored. Other vehicles are glycerin, syrup.
7. Syrups—nearly saturated solutions of a sugar, and may contain active medicinal agents.
8. Emulsions—mixtures of two immiscible liquids (usually water and an oil).
9. Gels—insoluble drugs in a semisolid form.

## Parenteral Route

Parenteral literally means any route other than the intestine. Common clinical meaning, however, is the route of injection.

Types of injection include the following:
1. Intradermal
2. Hypodermic (SC)
3. Intramuscular (IM)
4. Intravenous (IV)

Figure 1–5

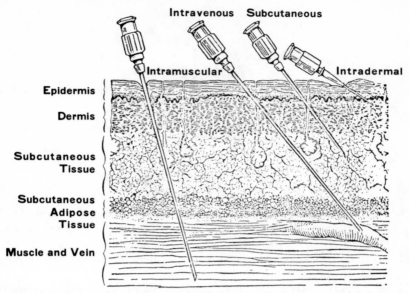

**Fig 1–5.**—Skin layers differentiating the types of injection given. (Adapted from Plein, J. D., and Plein, E. M.: *Fundamentals of Medication* [2d ed.; Hamilton, Ill.: Hamilton Press, Inc., 1974].)

5. Intra-arterial—into the artery. Drawing blood gases for an arterial sample involves placing a needle into an artery. This route is useful for treating the specific area perfused by the artery.
6. Intraspinal—injection through a vertebral interspace into the spinal subarachnoid space.
7. Epidural—injection through a vertebral interspace between the dura of the spinal cord and the periosteal lining of the spinal canal.
8. Intraperitoneal—inserting a needle or trocar into the peritoneal space. Frequently used for peritoneal dialysis.

"Drawing up" a dose for injection is usually from either an *ampule* or *vial.*

### Inhalation Route

An extremely important route for the respiratory therapist is the absorption of drugs in the vapor state or as a topical aerosol, by the alveoli and mucous membrane of the respiratory tract.

Common devices for inhalation of drugs include:

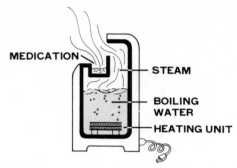

**Fig 1–6.**—Vaporizer, or steam inhaler.

1. Vaporizers—use heated water to form steam, the vehicle for carrying volatile drug solutions (Fig 1–6). These are less frequently used clinically.
2. Humidifiers—provide cold aerosol, usually water, by impeller nebulization.
3. Atomizers—essentially nebulizers without *any* baffles, using the Venturi principle (Fig 1–7). Frequently used for topical anesthesia in elective intubations.
4. Nebulizers—utilize a Venturi to mix two fluids, and a baffle to

**Fig 1–7.**—Atomizer.

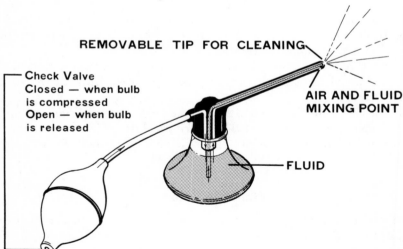

Inhalation Administration

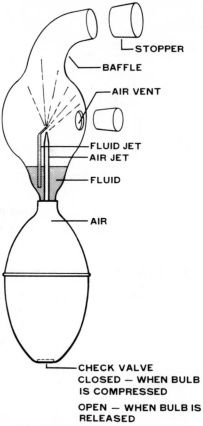

Fig 1–8.—Hand-powered nebulizer.

produce consistent particle size (Fig 1–8). This is the most common aerosol-producing device in respiratory therapy. Usually powered by compressed gas.
5. Inhalers—contain a relatively volatile medication embedded in some inert substance. The vapors are drawn into the nose by inhaling (Fig 1–9).
6. Mistometer aerosols—pressurized cartridges, or aerosol canlike devices. Usually powered by Freon-type gas to produce aerosol (Fig 1–10). Frequently abused by chronic respiratory patients.

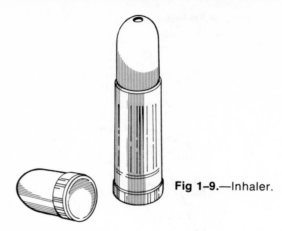

**Fig 1–9.**—Inhaler.

Usually contain bronchodilators. For further discussion of problems seen with mistometer delivery, see Chapter 4.

### Topical Route—Mucous Membranes

Topical application is often used in the nose, throat, or rectum, vagina, or ureter as a means of systemic effect because of the good absorption in these vascularized areas.
1. Lozenges—disks or flat squares of flavored medication which dissolve in the mouth.
2. Ophthalmic solutions—for the eye.
3. Nasal solutions—for the nose.
4. Otic solutions—for the ear.
5. Sublingual tablets—for absorption under the tongue.
6. Buccal tablets—to be placed between the teeth and cheek.
7. Suppositories—solid forms of medication prepared in a base (cacao butter, glycerinated gelatin, or polyethylene glycols) which will soften or dissolve at body temperature. Rectal, vaginal, or (rarely) urethral.

### Topical Route—Skin Application

Strictly a topical or local, rather than systemic, effect. Includes:
1. Powders.
2. Wet preparations—dressing, soaks, and baths.
3. Lotions—aqueous preparations which may be solutions, suspensions, or emulsions.

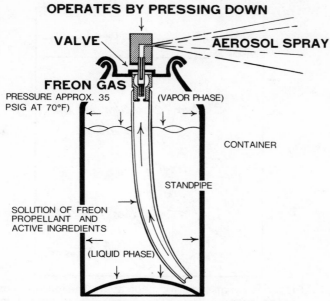

**Fig 1–10.**—Gas-powered aerosol cartridge.

4. Liniment—oily or alcoholic topical solutions, suspensions, or emulsions.
5. Ointments—semisolid preparations which may have anhydrous bases, emulsions of oil in water, or water-washable substances such as polyethylene glycols.
6. Creams—semisolid, less solid than ointments, with water-soluble or vanishing-cream base.
7. Pastes—stiff ointment-like preparations containing large quantities of powdered drugs such as zinc oxide or starch.
8. Jellies—viscous, semisolid preparations, usually made by hydrating gums. Lubricant, or vehicle.

## THE PRESCRIPTION

The prescription is the written order for a drug, along with any specific instructions for compounding, dispensing, and taking the drug.

This order may be written by a physician, osteopath, dentist, veterinarian, and others, but not chiropractors and opticians.

The detailed parts of a prescription are shown in Figure 1–11. It should be noted that both Latin and English, as well as metric and

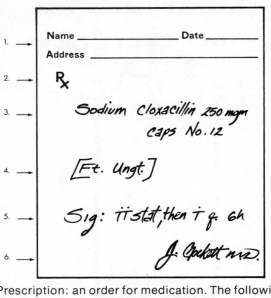

**Fig 1–11.**—Prescription: an order for medication. The following parts of the prescription can be seen: *1.* Patient's name, address, and date. *2.* Rx— "recipe" or "take thou." This directs the pharmacist to take the drugs listed and prepare the medication. This symbol is called the *superscription. 3.* The *inscription*—lists the names and quantities of the drugs. *4.* When applicable, this is the *subscription*, or directions to the pharmacist on preparing the medication. In many cases, with precompounded drugs, counting out the correct number is the only requirement. The directions here indicate that an ointment is to be made, which might be appropriate for certain medications. *5.* Sig—for signa meaning "write." The *transcription* or *signature*; the pharmacist writes this on the label of the medication as instructions to the patient. *6.* Name of the prescriber.

apothecary measures, have been used for drug orders. The directions (subscription; point 4 in Fig 1–11) to the pharmacist for mixing or compounding drugs have become less necessary with the advent of large pharmaceutical firms and their prepared drug products. The importance of these directions, however, is in no way diminished since misinterpretation is potentially lethal when dealing with drugs.

A list of the most common abbreviations seen with prescriptions is shown in Table 1–1. Most abbreviations are derived from the Latin, the mother tongue of medicine.

Since the Controlled Substances Act of 1971, a physician must include his/her registration number, given by the Drug Enforcement Administration (and usually termed a *DEA registration number*), when prescribing narcotics or controlled substances. Any licensed physician may apply for such a number.

## TABLE 1–1.—ABBREVIATIONS USED IN PRESCRIPTIONS

| ABBREVIATION | MEANING | ABBREVIATION | MEANING |
|---|---|---|---|
| aa | of each | ou | both eyes |
| ac | before meals | part aeq | equal parts |
| ad | to, up to | pc | after meals |
| ad lib | as much as desired | pil | pill |
| alt hor | every other hour | placebo | I please |
| aq dest | distilled water | po | by mouth |
| bid | twice daily | prn | as needed |
| C, cong | gallon | pro rect | rectally |
| c̄ | with | pulv | powder |
| caps | capsule | q | every |
| cc | cubic centimeter | qh | every hour |
| dil | dilute | qid | 4 times daily |
| dtd | give such doses | qod | every other day |
| elix | elixir | qd | every day |
| emuls | emulsion | q2h | every 2 hours |
| et | and | q3h | every 3 hours |
| ext | extract | q4h | every 4 hours |
| ex aq | in water | qs | as much as required |
| fl or fld | fluid | qt | quart |
| ft | make | Px, Rx | take |
| gel | a gel, jelly | s̄ | without |
| gm | gram | SC | subcutaneous |
| gr | grain | sig | write |
| gtt | a drop | sol | solution |
| hs | at bedtime | solv | dissolve |
| HT | hypodermic tablet | sos | if needed (for one time) |
| IM | intramuscular | sp or spir | spirit |
| IV | intravenous | sp frumenti | whiskey |
| I & O | intake and output | s̄s̄ | half |
| L | liter | stat | immediately |
| lin | a liniment | syr | syrup |
| liq | liquid, solution | tab | tablet or tablets |
| lot | lotion | tid | 3 times daily |
| M | mix | tr, tinct | tincture |
| mist | mixture | ung, ungt | ointment |
| ml | milliliter | ut dict | as directed |
| nebul | a spray | vin | wine |
| non rep | not to be repeated | ℨ | dram |
| NPO | nothing by mouth | ♏ | minim |
| O | pint | ℥ | ounce |
| od | right eye | ℈ | scruple |
| ol | oil | | |
| os | left eye | | |

## MEDICATION TEACHING CARD

A convenient and efficient method of updating or reviewing one's knowledge of pharmacologic agents is through the use of drug cards. A brief synopsis of essential information can be listed on a 3 × 5 index card (Fig 1–12). Printed ready-made forms are also available, but development of one's own system of cards will probably lead to greater reinforcement and retention of knowledge most useful for daily clinical practice as well as board examinations.

## RESPIRATORY THERAPY PHARMACOLOGY—A COMPREHENSIVE OVERVIEW

One of the central themes of respiratory therapy has been care of the patient's airway, from acute emergency situations to chronic maintenance and rehabilitation. This theme has not only defined the field, including clinical responsibilities and equipment, but has proved definitive of that area known as respiratory therapy pharmacology. In particular, all of the drugs used in respiratory therapy can be considered as *bronchoactive*, with one purpose, *airway patency*, through two major modes of action:
1. Control/reduction of secretions;
2. Relaxation of bronchial smooth muscle.
The relatively small group of bronchoactive drugs directly used by the therapist might be categorized as follows:
1. Humidifiers
    Normal saline (0.9%)

**Fig 1–12.**—Example of a medication teaching card which can be easily prepared on a 3 × 5 index card.

```
┌─────────────────────────────────────────────────────────────┐
│                                                               │
│    DRUG NAME:    GENERIC _____  CLASS_____      │
│                  TRADE  _____                         │
│                                                               │
│    STRENGTH: _____   DOSAGE: _____            │
│                                                               │
│    MODE OF ACTION:                                            │
│    HAZARDS/CONTRAINDICATIONS:                                 │
│    INTERACTIONS:                                              │
│                                                               │
└─────────────────────────────────────────────────────────────┘
```

Half-normal saline (0.45%)
Distilled water
2. Bronchodilators
Epinephrine HCl 1:100
Racemic epinephrine (Micronefrin, Vaponefrin)
Isoproterenol 1:200 (Isuprel)
Isoproterenol and cyclopentamine (Aerolone)
Isoetharine with phenylephrine (Bronkosol)
Metaproterenol sulfate (Alupent, Metaprel)
Terbutaline sulfate (Bricanyl)
Salbutamol—not yet available
Atropine sulfate
Sch 1000 (ipratropium bromide)—not yet available
3. Mucolytics
Sodium bicarbonate 2%
Acetylcysteine (Mucomyst, Mucomyst-10)
Pancreatic dornase (Dornavac)—no longer available
4. Surface-active agents
Ethyl alcohol 30–50%
Tyloxapol (Alevaire)
Sodium ethasulfate (Tergemist)—no longer available
5. Corticosteroids
Dexamethasone sodium phosphate (Decadron Respihaler)
Beclomethasone dipropionate (Vanceril inhaler)
Triamcinolone acetonide—not yet available
6. Asthma prophylactic
Cromolyn sodium (Intal, Aarane)

All of the drugs just listed can be given by the aerosol route of administration, with the exception of terbutaline sulfate, which is supplied in tablet form or for subcutaneous injection. In addition to these classes of drugs, the respiratory therapist is very closely involved with other classes such as antibiotics, pH buffers, neuromuscular blocking agents, and expectorants and antitussives. Another class of drugs which the therapist may be dealing with or administering in the future is prostaglandins, which seem to have great potential for control of bronchial contraction when delivered by aerosol.

## REFERENCES

Ahlquist, R. P.: Study of adrenotropic receptors, Am. J. Physiol. 153:586, 1948.
Asperheim, M. K., and Eisenhauer, L. A.: *The Pharmacologic Basis of Patient Care* (2d ed.; Philadelphia: W. B. Saunders Co., 1973).
Aviado, D. M. (ed.): *Krantz and Carr's Pharmacologic Principles of Medical Practice* (8th ed.; Baltimore: Williams & Wilkins Co., 1972).

DeKornfeld, T. J.: *Pharmacology for Respiratory Therapy* (Sarasota, Fla.: Glenn Educational Medical Services, Inc., 1976).

DiPalma, J. R. (ed.): *Drill's Pharmacology in Medicine* (4th ed.; New York: McGraw-Hill Book Co., 1971).

Fields, L. J., Williams, T. J., and Garavaglia, M. M.: *Pharmacologic Review for Intensive Cardiopulmonary Therapy* (Sarasota, Fla.: Glenn Educational Medical Services, Inc., 1975).

Goodman, L. S., and Gilman, A.: *The Pharmacological Basis of Therapeutics* (5th ed.; New York: Macmillan, 1975).

Goth, A.: *Medical Pharmacology* (7th ed.; St. Louis: C. V. Mosby Co., 1974).

Lands, A. M., et al.: Differentiation of receptor systems activated by sympathomimetic amines, Nature 214:597, 1967.

Langley, J. N.: On the physiology of the salivary secretion. Part II, J. Physiol. 1:339, 1878.

Meyers, F. H., Jawetz, E., and Goldfien, A.: *Review of Medical Pharmacology* (4th ed.; Los Altos, Calif.: Lange Medical Publications, 1974).

Modell, W., Schild, H. O., and Wilson, A.: *Applied Pharmacology* (11th ed.; Philadelphia: W. B. Saunders Co., 1976).

Plein, J. D., and Plein, E. M.: *Fundamentals of Medication* (2d ed.; Hamilton, Ill.: Hamilton Press, Inc., 1974).

Saxton, D. F., and Walter, J. F.: *Programmed Instruction in Arithmetic, Dosages, and Solutions* (3d ed.; St. Louis: C. V. Mosby Co., 1974).

# CHAPTER 2

# Calculating Drug Dosages

ALTHOUGH use of the metric system is now becoming standardized in the United States, a total of three systems of weights and measures have been employed in pharmacology: the metric system, the apothecary system, and the avoirdupois system. Those who are responsible for administering medications will in most cases encounter metric scales in both drug dosage strengths and drug orders. For the sake of completeness, however, and as a future reference, all three systems of measure are presented, since they have been used in pharmacology calculations.

## THE METRIC SYSTEM

The metric system is based on the decimal system, using multiples or fractions of 10.

Primary units in the metric system are meter (length), liter (volume), and gram (weight).

Fractional parts of these primary units are expressed by adding Latin prefixes for sizes smaller than the primary unit, and Greek prefixes for sizes larger than the primary unit.

Decreasing prefixes (Latin):

$$micro = 1/1,000,000$$
$$milli = 1/1,000$$
$$centi = 1/100$$
$$deci = 1/10$$

Increasing prefixes (Greek):

$$deka = 10$$
$$hecto = 100$$
$$kilo = 1,000$$

### Metric Table of Length

| 10 millimeters | = 1 centimeter | 10 mm | = 1 cm |
|---|---|---|---|
| 10 centimeters | = 1 decimeter | 10 cm | = 1 dm |

23

| 10 decimeters | = 1 meter | 10 dm | = 1 m |
|---|---|---|---|
| 10 meters | = 1 dekameter | 10 m | = 1 Dm |
| 10 dekameters | = 1 hectometer | 10 Dm | = 1 Hm |
| 10 hectometers | = 1 kilometer | 10 Hm | = 1 km |

### Metric Table of Volume

| 10 milliliters | = 1 centiliter | 10 ml | = 1 cl |
|---|---|---|---|
| 10 centiliters | = 1 deciliter | 10 cl | = 1 dl |
| 10 deciliters | = 1 liter | 10 dl | = 1 L |
| 10 liters | = 1 dekaliter | 10 L | = 1 Dl |
| 10 dekaliters | = 1 hectoliter | 10 Dl | = 1 Hl |
| 10 hectoliters | = 1 kiloliter | 10 Hl | = 1 kl |

### Metric Table of Weight

| 1,000 micrograms (gammos) | = 1 milligram | 1,000 μg | = 1 mg |
|---|---|---|---|
| 10 milligrams | = 1 centigram | 10 mg | = 1 cg |
| 10 centigrams | = 1 decigram | 10 cg | = 1 dg |
| 10 decigrams | = 1 gram | 10 dg | = 1 gm |
| 10 grams | = 1 dekagram | 10 gm | = 1 Dg |
| 10 dekagrams | = 1 hectogram | 10 Dg | = 1 Hg |
| 10 hectograms | = 1 kilogram | 10 Hg | = 1 kg |

NOTE: The gram is defined as the weight of one milliliter of pure water at standard temperature and pressure. Under these conditions one gram of water and one milliliter of water are equal. This should not be used to convert from weight to volume, however, as a gram of liquid is *not always* equal to a milliliter of liquid, depending on the temperature, pressure, and nature of the substance.

## THE APOTHECARY SYSTEM

Unlike the metric system, units of measurement in the apothecary system are not consistent. These units also have characteristic symbols (see Table 1–1). In the tables that follow, the units are spelled out, for easy recognition.

Several conventions apply if apothecary measure is used.

1. If the abbreviation or symbol for a unit is used, then the amount *follows* the symbol and is written in small Roman numerals.

EXAMPLE:

2 grains is gr ii
6 drams is ℥ vi

2. Fractions are written as fractions, with the amount following the abbreviation. The exception to this rule is use of ʒ̄ʒ̄ instead of $1/2$.

EXAMPLE:

$1/2$ ounce is oz ʒ̄ʒ̄

$1/4$ grain is gr $1/4$

The apothecary weight and fluid (volume) measures are given in the following tables.

### Apothecary's Weight

| | |
|---|---|
| 20 grains | = 1 scruple |
| 3 scruples | = 1 dram |
| 8 drams | = 1 ounce |
| 12 ounces | = 1 pound |

### Apothecary's Fluid Measures

| | |
|---|---|
| 60 minims | = 1 fluid dram |
| 8 fluid drams | = 1 fluid ounce |
| 16 fluid ounces | = 1 pint |
| 2 pints | = 1 quart |
| 4 quarts | = 1 gallon |

## THE AVOIRDUPOIS SYSTEM

The avoirdupois system is used in commerce, as well as in calculating drug dosage by the weight of the patient. For example, bicarbonate administration is based on the patient's weight in kilograms. The avoirdupois system contains only *weight measurement*—not *volume.*

NOTE: The avoirdupois system uses the same terms as found in the apothecary system of weight; the grain, however, is the only unit identical in both systems. There are 12 ounces per pound apothecary, and 16 ounces per pound avoirdupois. Therefore 1 pound apothecary is 5,760 grains, while 1 pound avoirdupois is 7,000 grains.

### Avoirdupois Weight

| | |
|---|---|
| $437^{1}/_{2}$ grains | = 1 ounce |
| 16 ounces | = 1 pound |
| 7,000 grains | = 1 pound |

In addition to the three systems of measure noted, there exists a set of household measures, which are included in the list of equivalents.

## INTERSYSTEM CONVERSIONS

All drugs manufactured today in the United States should have metric units for dosage strengths and amounts. All orders for drugs should similarly utilize metric units. A list of approximate equivalents, however, is given to aid in conversion from one system to another, including to household measures. It is stressed that this set of equivalents is only *approximate,* but has been considered to be helpful clinically. Slightly different sets of equivalents can be found in different texts. For accurate drug administration, drug orders should always employ the units in which the drug is supplied by the manufacturer.

### Approximate Equivalents

#### Metric

1 milligram = 0.015 grain
1 gram     = 15 grains
1 kilogram = 2.2 pounds (avdp)
1 milliliter = 15 minims or 16 drops (gtt)

#### Apothecary

1 grain          = 60 milligrams
1 ounce (apoth)  = 30 grams
1 fl dram (apoth) = 4 milliliters
1 fl oz (apoth)  = 30 milliliters
1 pint           = 500 milliliters
1 quart          = 1,000 milliliters
1 gallon         = 4,000 milliliters
1 minim          = 1 drop (gtt)

#### Avoirdupois

1 pound = 454 grams
1 ounce = 28.3 grams

#### Household Equivalents

1 teaspoon    = 5 milliliters     = 1¼ fl dram
1 tablespoon = 15 milliliters    = 4 fl drams
1 cup         = 240 milliliters   = 8 fl ounces
1 pint        = 500 milliliters
1 quart       = 1,000 milliliters

Problems on conversion from metric-apothecary-avoirdupois systems can be found in Chapter 14.

## DRUG DOSAGE CALCULATION

Once the therapist is able to freely convert within the metric system, and between the metric and apothecary systems, it is possible to begin calculating drug dosages.

In general, such calculations will be of two types:

1. Those involving fluids, tablets, or capsules of a given strength, e.g., 5 mg per milliliter, and,

2. Those involving solutions of a percentage strength.

Since there are definite conventions regarding solutions, and since solutions for aerosol delivery are the primary dosage form for respiratory therapy, they are treated separately, in detail.

## CALCULATING DOSAGES FROM PREPARED-STRENGTH LIQUIDS, TABLETS, AND CAPSULES

When using a prepared-strength liquid, tablet, or capsule, you are always trying to determine *how much* liquid, or *how many* tablets or capsules are needed to give the strength of the drug ordered. For example, if one aspirin tablet contains 5 grains of aspirin and you want to give 2.5 grains, you immediately realize that *half* a tablet must be given.

The simplest, and therefore probably the most accurate or error-free, method of calculation when using a vial of a prepared-strength drug (or tablet or capsule) involves two steps at most:

1. Convert to consistent units of measure;

2. Set up a straightforward proportion:

$$\frac{\text{original drug strength}}{\text{amount}} = \frac{\text{desired drug strength}}{\text{amount}}$$

or,

original strength : amount :: desired strength : amount

In step 1, this conversion may be from apothecary to metric, or vice versa (if an apothecary dosage strength has been ordered, and is thus the desired strength), or from grams to milligrams *within* the metric system.

For example, if you have oxytetracycline tablets, each 250 milligram strength, and you need 0.5 grams of the drug, either convert 250 mg to 0.25 gm, or 0.5 gm to 500 mg.

Once the units are consistent, set up the proportion to find the unknown, which is how many tablets are needed to deliver the desired dose to the patient. Using the formula just given:

$$\text{original drug strength} = 250 \text{ mg}$$
$$\text{amount} = \text{tablet}$$
$$\text{desired drug strength} = 0.5 \text{ gm} = 500 \text{ mg}$$
$$\text{amount} = \text{unknown}$$
$$\frac{250 \text{ mg}}{1 \text{ tablet}} = \frac{500 \text{ mg}}{X \text{ tablet}}$$
$$500 \times 1 = 250 \times X$$
$$X = \frac{500}{250}$$
$$= 2 \text{ tablets}$$

While this calculation is simple and can be performed mentally, others may require calculation for the sake of accuracy.

EXAMPLE 1: You have 120 mg of phenobarbital in 30 ml of phenobarbital elixir. How many ml of elixir will you use to give a 15 mg dose?

$$\frac{120 \text{ mg (original strength)}}{30 \text{ ml (amount)}} = \frac{15 \text{ mg (desired strength)}}{X \text{ (amount)}}$$
$$\frac{120 \text{ mg}}{30 \text{ ml}} = \frac{15 \text{ mg}}{X}$$
$$120 \times X = 450$$
$$X = 3.75 \text{ ml}$$

Simplification is possible, such as reducing 120 mg/30 ml to 4 mg/1 ml. Then, knowing that there are 4 mg in every ml, simply divide 4 mg/ml into 15 mg, to determine how many ml are needed. Often, reducing a fluid to its dosage strength per *one* milliliter allows quick mental computation of the dose. Caution and care, however, should be observed in the initial reduction. An error at that point causes a subsequent dosage error. *Do not hesitate to write out a calculation:* in a busy, clinical setting, a patient's well-being should take precedence over a therapist's mathematical pride!

There are other ways of expressing the same proportion, such as:

original strength : desired strength :: original amount : desired amount

As long as extremes, and means, are each multiplied together, the correct answer will result. If one arrangement is intuitively clearer, then that is preferable for the person using it.

EXAMPLE 2: Scopolamine HBr $^1/_{60}$ grain is ordered; you have 0.4 mg tablets; how many tablets would you use to prepare the dose?

a. Convert $^1/_{60}$ grain to milligrams:

$$1 \text{ grain } = 60 \text{ mg}$$
$$^1/_{60} \text{ gr} \times 60 \text{ mg/gr} = 1 \text{ mg}$$
$$\text{so, } ^1/_{60} \text{ gr} = 1 \text{ mg}$$

b. $\dfrac{0.4 \text{ mg strength}}{1 \text{ tablet}} = \dfrac{1.0 \text{ mg strength}}{X \text{ tablets}}$

$$0.4X = 1$$
$$X = \dfrac{1}{0.4}$$
$$= 2^1/_2 \text{ tablets}$$

NOTE: Some drugs are manufactured in units rather than in grams, grains, or drams. Examples are penicillin, insulin, and heparin, or pancreatic dornase, which was manufactured in 50,000 units per milliliter. Solving dosage problems for these drugs is exactly the same as for the other dosage units previously mentioned.

EXAMPLE 3: To give 75,000 units of pancreatic dornase, you would set up the following proportions:

$$100,000 \text{ units} : 2 \text{ ml} :: 75,000 \text{ units} : X \text{ ml}$$
$$X = 1.5 \text{ ml}$$

Problems of dosage calculation with prepared-strength drugs can be found in Chapter 14.

## CALCULATING DOSAGES FROM PERCENTAGE-STRENGTH SOLUTIONS

Since the respiratory therapist deals almost exclusively with the inhalation route and therefore aerosols, solutions and percentage strengths are fundamental to his/her work with drugs.

A *solution* contains a *solute* which is dissolved in a *solvent,* giving a homogeneous mixture.

The *strength* of a solution is expressed in percentage of solute to total solvent and solute. *Percentage means:* parts of the active ingredient (solute) in a preparation contained in 100 parts of the total preparation (solute *and* solvent).

## Types of Percentage Preparations

*Weight to weight:* Percentage in weight (W/W) expresses the number of grams of a drug or active ingredient in 100 grams of a mixture.

W/W: grams per 100 grams of mixture

*Weight to volume:* Percentage may be expressed for the number of grams of a drug or active ingredient in 100 milliliters of a mixture.

W/V: grams per 100 milliliters of mixture

*Volume to volume:* Percentage volume in volume (V/V) expresses the number of milliliters of a drug or active ingredient in 100 milliliters of a mixture.

V/V: milliliters per 100 milliliters of mixture

NOTE: Calculating percentage strengths of solutions by *either* weight of a drug in grams, *or* by volume of a drug in milliliters, and taking percentages of grams to milliliters, is based on, or allowed because:

$$1 \text{ gm } H_2O = 1 \text{ ml } H_2O \text{ at STP}$$

### SOLUTIONS BY RATIO

Frequently when diluting a medication for use in an aerosol or IPPB treatment, a solute to solvent *ratio* is given, e.g., isoproterenol 1:200 or Bronkosol 1:8.

RATIO BY GRAMS : MILLILITERS: In the isoproterenol example, what is indicated is:

1 gram per 200 ml of solution = 0.5% strength

Other examples:

epinephrine 1:100 = 1% strength
epinephrine 1:1,000 = 0.1% strength

Generally: grams per milliliters, or grams : milliliters, are the intended units.

RATIO BY SIMPLE PARTS: In the Bronkosol example, actual parts medication to parts solvent is indicated:

1:8 = 1 part to 8 parts

or, 1 ml to 8 ml ratio, which is the same as:

$1/4$ ml to 2 ml.

However, part-to-part ratios do *not* indicate actual amounts or specific units, although usually milliliters : milliliters is meant. It is assumed you know Bronkosol is given in $1/4$ ml doses, not 1 ml doses, as far as the absolute amount is concerned. Ratio by simple parts is not precise unless the absolute amount of the drug is specified and the original strength of the drug to be used is known.

## NOTE ON MIXING SOLUTIONS

One determines the amount of active ingredient needed for the percentage strength desired, and then adds enough solvent to "top off" to the *total* solution amount needed. When ordering a solution this is indicated by "qs", or "quantity sufficient," for the total needed.

For example, to obtain 30 ml of 3% procaine HCl, we calculate 0.9 ml of the active ingredient, and water qs for 30 ml of solution.

One does not merely give the difference between solute and total solution (30 ml − 0.9 ml = 29.1 ml) because certain solutes can change volume, e.g., alcohol "shrinks" in water.

### Solving Percentage and Solution Problems

For solutions when the active ingredient itself is pure (undiluted, 100% strength), the following statements are easily used:

$$\text{percentage strength} = \frac{\text{solute (in grams or ml)}}{\text{total amount (solute and solvent)}}$$

or, alternatively, a ratio format,

$$\frac{\text{amount of solute}}{\text{total amount}} = \frac{\text{amount of solute}}{100 \text{ parts (gm or ml)}}$$

When the active ingredient, or solute, itself is less than pure, the following equation may be used to calculate the amount of solute needed.

$$\text{percentage strength} = \frac{(\text{dilute solute}) \times (\text{percentage strength of solute})}{\text{total amount of solution}}$$

In brief, the solute (active ingredient) times the percentage strength of the solute gives the amount of pure active ingredient in the total solution (solute plus solvent).

Equation 3 adds only one modification to the formula given in equation 1. This is to multiply the dilute solute by its actual percentage strength, with the result indicating the amount of active ingredient at a 100% (pure) strength. For example, 10 milliliters of 10% solute *means* you have 1 milliliter of pure solute. Put another way, you would need 10 ml of dilute solute to have 1 ml of pure solute (active ingredient). When used in equation 3, the unknown is usually how much of the dilute solute, or active ingredient, is needed in the total solution to give the desired strength. This is illustrated in example 2.

EXAMPLE 1—UNDILUTED ACTIVE INGREDIENT: How many milligrams of active ingredient are there in 2 ml of 1:200 isoproterenol?

percentage strength = 1:200 = 0.5% = 0.005
total amount of solution = 2 ml
active ingredient = $X$

$$0.005 = \frac{X \text{ gm}}{2 \text{ ml}}$$

$$X \text{ gm} = 0.005 \times 2$$

$$X = 0.01 \text{ gm}$$

Converting 0.01 grams to milligrams gives 10 mg. In 2 ml of 1:200 solution there are 10 mg.

EXAMPLE 2—DILUTED ACTIVE INGREDIENT: How much 10% procaine HCl is needed to prepare 1 fluid ounce of 3% procaine HCl solution to use as a local for an arterial puncture?

First convert 1 fluid ounce apothecary to metric:

$$1 \text{ fl ounce} = 30 \text{ ml}$$

Then, percentage strength (needed) = 3% = 0.03
total solution = 30 ml
active ingredient = $X$
percentage strength of active ingredient = 10% = 0.10

Substitute:

$$0.03 = \frac{X \times 0.10}{30 \text{ ml}}$$

$$X = \frac{0.03 \times 30}{0.10}$$

= 9 ml of the 10% strength procaine, mixed with enough water to give a total of 30 ml solution.

Additional examples and practice problems on solutions and percentages can be found in Chapter 14.

## SUMMARY OF METHODS FOR SOLVING PERCENTAGE PROBLEMS

### Solutions and Percentages

$$W:W \ \% = \frac{grams}{100 \ grams}$$

$$W:V \ \% = \frac{grams}{100 \ milliliters} \left. \right\} \ \% = \frac{solute}{total \ solution}$$

$$V:V \ \% = \frac{milliliters}{100 \ milliliters}$$

1. Convert to metric units and decimal expressions.
2. Substitute knowns in the appropriate % equation.
3. Express answer in units or system requested.

Remember the definition of percentage strength:

percentage = parts (gm, ml) per 100 parts

*You must use grams or milliliters in the percentage equation.*
NOTE: 1:200 = 1 gram per 200 milliliters.

## SOLUTIONS: DEFINITIONS AND TERMS

*Solution:* physically homogeneous mixture of two or more substances (liquid).
*Isotonic solutions:* have equal osmotic pressures.
*Buffer solution:* aqueous solution able to resist changes of pH with addition of acid/base.

### STRENGTH OF SOLUTIONS

*Normal (N) solution:* one gram-equivalent weight (GEW) of solute per liter of solution.
*Molar solution:* one mole of solute per liter of solution.
*Molal solution:* one mole of solute per 1,000 grams of solvent.
*Osmole solution:* molarity × number of particles per molecule.
*Osmolar solution:* one osmole per liter of solution.
*Osmolal solution:* one osmole per kilogram of solvent.
EXAMPLE—NORMAL VS PHYSIOLOGIC (ISOTONIC) SALINE:
    1 normal solution NaCl

NaCl – GEW      = 58.5 gm
∴ 1 N solution     = 58.5 gm/L, or
                   = 5.85 gm/100 ml
                   = 5.85% solution
Physiologic saline = 0.9% NaCl (isotonic to body fluid)
                   = 0.9 gm/100 ml
1 ml              = 0.009 gm NaCl

The 0.9% saline solution is isotonic to body fluid, and is usually termed "normal saline." This is not the same strength as a normal solution of NaCl.

## REFERENCES

Carr, J. J., McElroy, N. L., and Carr, B. L.: How to solve dosage problems in one easy lesson, Am. J. Nurs. 76:1934, 1976.

McDermid, G. L.: Calculating the amount of solute in a solution, Respir. Care 21:861, 1976.

Plein, J. D., and Plein, E. M.: *Fundamentals of Medication* (2d ed.; Hamilton, Ill.: Hamilton Press, Inc., 1974).

Richardson, L. I., and Richardson, J. K.: *The Mathematics of Drugs and Solutions with Clinical Applications* (New York: McGraw-Hill Book Co., 1976).

Saxton, D. F., and Walter, J. F.: *Programmed Instruction in Arithmetic, Dosages, and Solutions* (3d ed.; St. Louis: C. V. Mosby Co., 1974).

# CHAPTER 3

# The Central and Peripheral Nervous System

THE BEST APPROACH to understanding principles of drug action is through a clear, well-organized grasp of the central and peripheral nervous system, since numerous drugs in respiratory care exert their effects by altering this system.

The basic organization of the nervous system can be outlined as follows:

Central nervous system $\begin{cases} \text{Brain} \\ \text{Spinal cord} \end{cases}$

Peripheral nervous system $\begin{cases} \text{Sensory (afferent)} \\ \text{Motor (efferent)} \\ \text{Autonomic nervous system} \\ \quad \text{Parasympathetic branch} \\ \quad \text{Sympathetic branch} \end{cases}$

Figure 3–1 is a functional, but not anatomically accurate, diagram of the central and peripheral nervous system.

Impulses to the brain (afferent) from sensory receptors, and from the brain (efferent) to skeletal muscle are conveyed by a sequence of electrical and chemical means, which will be examined in detail for each junction of the system. Very generally, the sensory input, from heat, light, pressure, and pain receptors, as well as the skeletal muscle motor functions, are largely under conscious, voluntary control. The sensory and motor branches are also known in combination as the somatic system.

Neither the motor nor the sensory branches have synapses outside of the spinal cord before reaching the muscle or sensory receptor site. This is in contrast to the synapses occurring in the sympathetic and parasympathetic divisions of the autonomic system. The additional synapses of the autonomic system offer potential sites for drug effect, besides the terminal, neuroeffector sites.

35

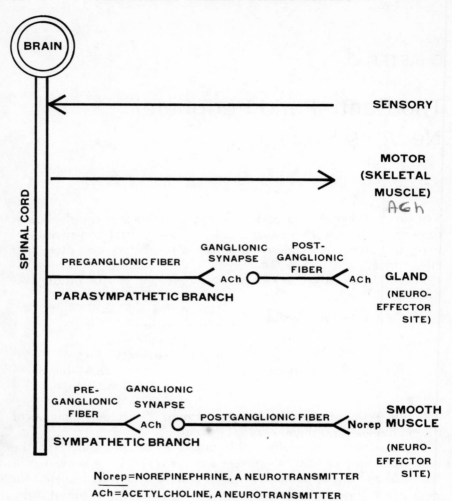

**Fig 3-1.**—A functional diagram of the central and peripheral nervous system, indicating the somatic branches (*sensory, motor*) and the autonomic branches (*sympathetic, parasympathetic*), with their synapses and neurotransmitters. (From Rau, J. L.: Respir. Care 22:263, 1977. Used by permission.)

It should be noted that the neurotransmitter at the motor (skeletal muscle) sites is acetylcholine, which is the same for the parasympathetic branch and all ganglionic synapses. The motor, or efferent, division is of great importance when considering neuromuscular blocking agents.

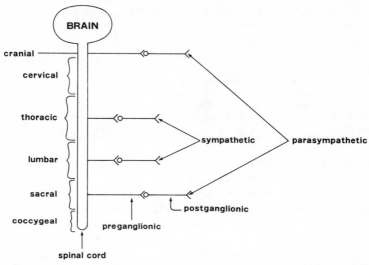

**Fig 3–2.**—Anatomical description of *parasympathetic* and *sympathetic* branches. This can be contrasted with the functionally organized diagram in Figure 3–1.

## AUTONOMIC NERVOUS SYSTEM

The autonomic nervous system is the involuntary, unconscious control mechanism of the body, sometimes said to control vegetative functions. It is divided into the parasympathetic and sympathetic branches, which maintain a balance of opposing effects on the body's smooth muscle, such as the myocardium, viscera (GI tract, stomach), and glands (lacrimal, salivary, mucosal).

### Parasympathetic Branch

The parasympathetic branch arises from the craniosacral portions of the spinal cord, and consists of two neurons: a preganglionic fiber leading from the cord to the ganglionic synapse outside the cord; and a postganglionic fiber from the ganglionic synapse to the gland or smooth muscle being innervated (Fig 3–2).

The parasympathetic branch has good specificity with the postganglionic fiber arising very near the effector site (gland, smooth muscle). This is a discrete system, whose effects are listed in Table 3–1.

### PARASYMPATHETIC NEUROTRANSMITTER

Nervous impulses are conducted by electrical and chemical means. Chemical transmission of the impulse occurs at synapses, and can be

TABLE 3–1.—PARASYMPATHETIC EFFECTS

| SITE | EFFECT |
|------|--------|
| Heart | Slows rate of SA node via vagus (X cranial) nerve |
| Bronchioles | Constricts |
| Bronchial mucus glands | Stimulates to secrete |
| Lacrimal, salivary, sweat | Increases secretion |
| Coronary, pulmonary | Vasodilation |
| Urinary bladder | Detrusor contracts, trigone and sphincter relax |
| Intestines | Increases motility, relaxes sphincters |

understood by considering the mode of action of acetylcholine at the parasympathetic effector site (Fig 3–3). Such chemicals are termed *neurotransmitters* or *neurohormones*.

Vesicles containing acetylcholine (ACh) are present in the end of the nerve fiber. The electrical nerve impulse releases ACh, formerly synthesized and stored, which attaches to receptors on the postsynaptic membrane. In somatic motor nerve endings, membrane permeability to Na$^+$ and K$^+$ is altered, depolarizing or "firing" the cell.

**Fig 3–3.**—Storage, release, and inactivation of the parasympathetic neurotransmitter, *acetylcholine.*

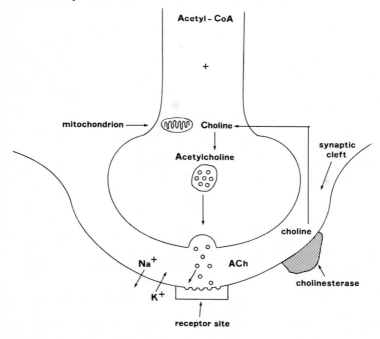

Acetylcholine is inactivated through hydrolysis by cholinesterase enzymes.

A similar event occurs in both the parasympathetic and sympathetic branches, at the ganglionic synapse and the effector site.

Acetylcholine is the neurotransmitter at motor nerve endings, and *all* autonomic synapses *except* the sympathetic effector site. Here the transmitter is usually considered to be norepinephrine, although this model does not satisfy all results obtainable. Some have postulated that isoproterenol is the sympathetic neurotransmitter, or that isoproterenol must be present for the norepinephrine to be effective.

Atropine, similar in structure to ACh, can *block* the transmission of the parasympathetic impulse by occupying the neuroeffector receptor site. This is termed competitive *inhibition,* and atropine is a *parasympatholytic.* A drug such as neostigmine facilitates parasympathetic and somatic nerve transmission by destroying cholinesterase. This drug is a *parasympathomimetic,* and termed *indirect acting* since it does not directly fire the receptor. Curare (*d*-tubocurarine) blocks motor nerve impulses, because its structure is also similar to ACh and competitively inhibits ACh to paralyze the muscles. Curare does not block parasympathetic transmission, selectively attaching to the motor nerve ends.

## SYMPATHETIC BRANCH

The sympathetic branch arises from the thoracolumbar portion of the spinal cord, has a short preganglionic and a long postganglionic fiber, with acetylcholine as the ganglionic neurotransmitter, and norepinephrine as the neurotransmitter at the neuroeffector site. Effects are listed in Table 3–2.

### TABLE 3–2.—SYMPATHETIC EFFECTS

| SITE | EFFECT |
| --- | --- |
| Heart | $\beta_1$, ↑ rate, conduction, force |
| Bronchial muscle | $\beta_2$, dilates, relaxes |
| Coronary and skeletal blood vessels | $\beta$, relax |
| Pulmonary and cerebral blood vessels | $\alpha$ and $\beta$, contract/relax* |
| Peripheral (dermal) blood vessel | $\alpha$, constricts |
| Sweat glands | $\alpha$, increases secretion |

*When alpha and beta receptors are equally distributed, the physiologic effect depends on which receptor type is more stimulated by a given drug. For example, norepinephrine will tend to cause vasoconstriction, because of greater alpha stimulation; isoproterenol will cause vasodilation, with little alpha effect (constriction); epinephrine may cause no net effect since equal alpha and beta stimulation will cancel each other.

The sympathetic system is the site of much pharmacologic manipulation in respiratory therapy, and offers a certain amount of complexity. The synapse at the effector site seems to be functionally similar to that of the parasympathetic. However, instead of inactivation by enzymes, re-uptake of the transmitter is most important for termination of the impulse, with catechol-$O$-methyltransferase (COMT) and monoamine oxidase (MAO) serving to metabolize any remaining norepinephrine (Fig 3–4).

In somewhat more detail, the sequence of production, storage, release, and inactivation of norepinephrine at the sympathetic effector site can be visualized in Figure 3–5.

Phenylalanine is converted to tyrosine by a hydroxylase enzyme, which in turn converts tyrosine to dopa. Dopa is changed to dopamine by dopa decarboxylase; dopamine then converts to norepinephrine, by action of dopamine-β. Norepinephrine is a precursor to epinephrine. This sequence may end with dopamine, norepinephrine, or epinephrine at actual sites.

Termination of the impulse at the neuroeffector site is primarily through re-uptake of the neurotransmitter. However, excess transmitter in the nerve terminal can be destroyed by MAO, and COMT can inactivate the transmitter in the synaptic cleft.

Sympathetic neuroeffector sites have been differentiated according to a spectrum of effects elicited by different drugs.

In 1948, Ahlquist distinguished *alpha-* and *beta-*sympathetic receptors on the basis of these differing responses to phenylephrine, norepinephrine, epinephrine, and isoproterenol.

Alpha receptors: generally *excite,* with the exception of the intestine, where relaxation occurs.

Beta receptors: generally *relax,* with the exception of the heart, where stimulation occurs.

From these early studies certain sites are considered as alpha, e.g., peripheral blood vessels, while others are designated beta, such as

**Fig 3–4.**—Detailed diagram of the sympathetic branch of the autonomic nervous system.

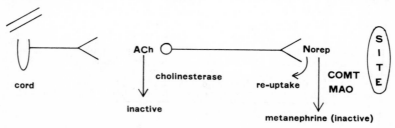

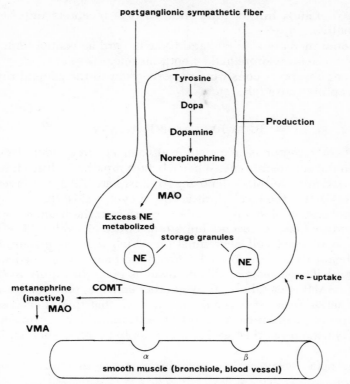

**Fig 3–5.**—Storage, release, and inactivation of the sympathetic neurotransmitter, *norepinephrine*.

bronchial smooth muscle. Drug activity of sympathetic stimulants (sympathomimetics) ranges along the spectrum seen in Figure 3–6.

As illustrated in Figure 3–6, phenylephrine is one of the purest alpha stimulants, and isoproterenol is an almost pure beta stimulant. It is stressed that "pure" reactions do not occur with any drug; i.e., even phenylephrine may affect other sites. Epinephrine stimulates both alpha and beta sites equally, but norepinephrine has more of an alpha than beta effect.

**Fig 3–6.**—Spectrum of activity of common sympathomimetics, ranging from alpha to beta stimulants.

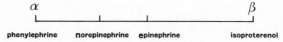

In 1967, Lands further differentiated beta receptors into beta-one and beta-two.

Beta-one: increases the rate and force of cardiac contraction.

Beta-two: relaxes bronchial smooth muscle.

Beta-one receptors constitute the exception to the general rule that beta receptors cause relaxation.

## BETA-RECEPTOR PATHWAY

The beta receptor is associated with an enzyme, adenyl cyclase, found in the cell membrane. When a beta-sympathetic drug attaches to the enzyme, intracellular adenosine triphosphate (ATP) is converted to cyclic AMP. It is the level of intracellular cyclic AMP that is responsible for relaxation of smooth muscle, whether in the bronchioles or in the blood vessels. A second important effect of cyclic AMP is the inhibition of mast cell degranulation which releases histamine and other chemicals causing bronchoconstriction and mucosal edema (see Chapter 9). The schema of this pathway is given in Figure 3–7.

Cyclic AMP is metabolized by another enzyme, phosphodiesterase, to an inactive form. It is interesting to note that this offers a second alternative to increasing cyclic AMP levels: inhibition of phosphodiesterase. The xanthine theophylline (aminophylline), is such an inhibitor.

When beta receptors become unresponsive to stimulation, *beta*

**Fig 3–7.**—The beta-receptor pathway. The beta receptor is considered to be the enzyme adenyl cyclase in the cell membrane, which, in combination with epinephrine or other catecholamines, catalyzes the conversion of *ATP* to *cyclic AMP*.

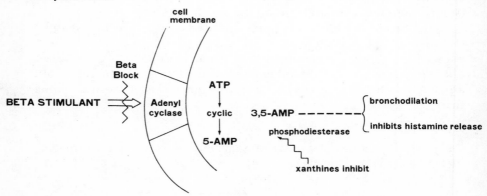

### TABLE 3–3.—AUTONOMIC EFFECTS IN THE CARDIOPULMONARY SYSTEM

| | PARASYMPATHETIC | SYMPATHETIC |
|---|---|---|
| **Lungs** | | |
| Bronchial smooth muscle | Constricts | $\beta_2$, relaxes (dilates) |
| Circulation | Vasodilation | $\alpha$ and $\beta$ |
| Bronchial mucus glands | Vagus, ↑ secretion | — |
| **Heart** | | |
| Atrium and A-V node | ↓ rate and force | $\beta_1$ { ↑force and conduction |
| Ventricle | — | { ↑rate & force |
| **Systemic circulation** | | |
| Peripheral (dermal) | Vasodilation | $\alpha$, constricts |
| Skeletal muscle | — | $\beta$, dilates |
| Coronary | — | $\beta$, dilates |
| Cerebral | — | $\alpha$ and $\beta$, contract/relax |

*blockade* is said to exist. As a physiologic occurrence, the cause or causes of this are not known. However, the same blockade can be induced pharmacologically with a beta-blocking drug such as propranolol (Inderal). A comprehensive summary of autonomic effects is shown in Table 3–3.

## TERMINOLOGY OF DRUGS AFFECTING THE AUTONOMIC NERVOUS SYSTEM

The terms that follow have been used to categorize autonomic drugs.

*Parasympathomimetic (cholinergic):* an agent causing stimulation of the parasympathetic nervous system.

*Parasympatholytic (anticholinergic):* an agent blocking or inhibiting effects of the parasympathetic nervous system.

*Sympathomimetic (adrenergic):* an agent causing stimulation of the sympathetic nervous system. Such agents are alpha stimulants (phenylephrine), beta stimulants (isoproterenol), beta-two stimulants (isoetharine), or alpha and beta stimulants (epinephrine).

*Sympatholytic (antiadrenergic):* an agent blocking or inhibiting the effect of the sympathetic nervous system.

Drugs are also categorized according to either their muscarinic or nicotinic effect upon the autonomic nervous system.

MUSCARINIC EFFECT: Alkaloid muscarine exerts effects similar to those of acetylcholine (ACh) at the parasympathetic effector sites; it affects smooth muscles, cardiac muscle, and exocrine glands. There is no effect on ganglionic or skeletal muscle sites. Therefore, effects of ACh on the parasympathetic sites are termed muscarinic; certain drugs such as neostigmine (Prostigmin) or edrophonium (Tensilon) which are indirect-acting parasympathomimetics (anticholinesterases) stimulate these sites. Secretions from exocrine glands such as the salivary, lacrimal, and bronchial can be an inconvenience when caring for a patient's airway. Therefore, when these drugs are used to reverse the effects of curare (a nondepolarizing neuromuscular blocker) on skeletal muscle, their additional *muscarinic* effect on the glands (also innervated by ACh) is blocked by atropine, a parasympatholytic. Atropine of course only blocks the autonomic effects of the anticholinesterase—not the skeletal muscle effect which reverses the curare.

NICOTINIC EFFECT: Nicotine affects the other two sites at which ACh works; it affects the ganglia and neuromuscular synapses. Thus the effects of ACh on these sites is termed nicotinic.

In summary,

*Muscarinic* is the effect of ACh on parasympathetic effector sites (smooth muscle, cardiac muscle, and exocrine glands).

*Nicotinic* is the effect of ACh on ganglionic and neuromuscular synapses.

## UNIFIED THEORY OF AUTONOMIC CONTROL IN LUNG

Much recent research has indicated that the parasympathetic and sympathetic branches balance each other to preserve normal bronchial patency and tone. In brief, it is thought that the parasympathetic and alpha-sympathetic effect is to tighten and constrict bronchiolar smooth muscle, while beta-sympathetic discharge opposes this with a relaxing effect (Fig 3–8). The *net* effect is tone: a tracheobronchial tree that is neither flaccid and lifeless nor tightly contracted.

Smooth muscle is not normally completely flaccid, just as skeletal muscle is not. In skeletal muscle, cutting neural innervation does not just relax the muscle, but causes it to be toneless—as seen with paraplegics. Muscle will actually atrophy. These differences of tonelessness and constriction versus normal tone can be visualized in Figure 3–9.

It is further thought that the effects of the autonomic system normally causing bronchial tone are mediated intracellularly through cyclic AMP, previously discussed in the section entitled "Beta-

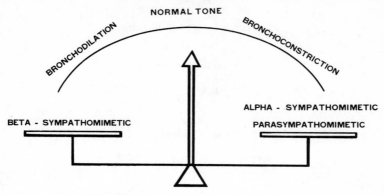

NORMAL TONE

BRONCHODILATION

BRONCHOCONSTRICTION

ALPHA - SYMPATHOMIMETIC

PARASYMPATHOMIMETIC

BETA - SYMPATHOMIMETIC

BALANCED AUTONOMIC CONTROL OF THE LUNG

**Fig 3–8.**—A graphic representation of the interplay of alpha-, beta-, and parasympathetic innervation in the bronchial tree. (From Rau, J. L.: Respir. Care 22:263, 1977. Used by permission.)

Receptor Pathway," and its counterpart, cyclic GMP. The comprehensive view of this hypothesis is presented in Figure 3–10.

ALPHA STIMULATION: results in a decrease in tissue cyclic AMP, leading to an imbalance of cyclic GMP.

BETA STIMULATION: results in an increase in cyclic AMP.

PARASYMPATHETIC STIMULATION: results in an increase in cyclic GMP.

The importance of the autonomic system for pulmonary pathology is evident when the biologic activity of these nucleotides is considered: Cyclic AMP

1. Relaxes smooth muscle to cause bronchodilation.
2. Inhibits mast cell degranulation which can release histamine to

**Fig 3–9.**—The differences in bronchoconstriction, bronchial relaxation, and normal bronchial muscle tone.

smooth muscle

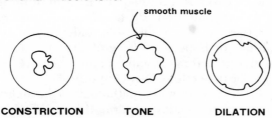

CONSTRICTION          TONE          DILATION

**GENERAL SCHEME OF**

**NERVOUS CONTROL IN LUNG**

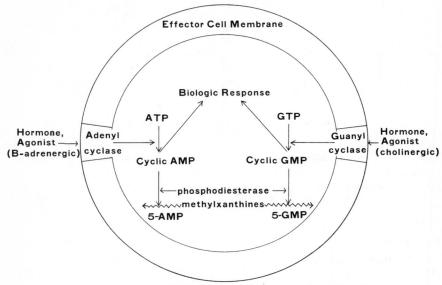

Cyclic **AMP** - biologic response = bronchodilation
Cyclic **GMP** - biologic response = bronchoconstriction

**Fig 3–10.**—A comprehensive view of autonomic effects mediated through the intracellular nucleotides, *cyclic AMP* and *cyclic GMP*. (From Rau, J. L.: Respir. Care 22:263, 1977. Used by permission.)

cause bronchoconstriction, secretions, and mucosal edema. This is the pathologic mechanism in extrinsic allergic (antigen-mediated) asthma (see Chapter 9).

Cyclic GMP

1. Contracts smooth muscle to cause bronchoconstriction.
2. Enhances mast cell release of histamine and other bronchoconstricting mediators.

This dramatic view offers a unified mechanism of bronchoconstriction, whether due to pollution, dust, aerosols, exercise, anxiety, or allergy. Rather than a simple beta-blockade theory to explain an intrinsic irritability or hypersensitivity of the bronchi, such as with intrinsic, non-allergic asthma, a more comprehensive theory of biochemical balance at the cellular level is proposed.

In addition to illuminating the pathology of bronchoconstriction, this view has offered alternatives in drug therapy. To block bronchoconstriction, one should be able to utilize the following:

*Beta sympathomimetics:* This is the traditional class of drugs, e.g., isoproterenol, many of which are used in respiratory care. *Effect*—increased cyclic AMP.

*Alpha sympatholytics:* If alpha stimulation decreases cyclic AMP, blocking alpha receptors should prevent a decrease. This has been attempted using phentolamine (an alpha blocker) with some success with chronic asthmatics. *Effect*—blocks decrease of cyclic AMP.

*Parasympatholytics:* This class of drugs, e.g., atropine, should block any increase in cyclic GMP, allowing a relative rise in cyclic AMP to cause bronchodilation. *Effect*—blocks the rise of cyclic GMP.

These three types of drugs, used singly or in combination, have given new possibilities in treatment, as well as new understanding of the causes of pulmonary disease.

Because of the experimental aspect of many of these concepts, an extensive bibliography is included to allow one interested in these new developments to extend his or her knowledge beyond the scope of these brief remarks.

## REFERENCES

Ahlquist, R. P.: Study of adrenotropic receptors, Am. J. Physiol. 153:586, 1948.

Austen, K. F.: A Review of Immunological, Biochemical and Pharmacological Factors in the Release of Chemical Mediators from the Human Lung, in Austen, K. F., and Lichtenstein, L. M. (eds.): *Asthma: Physiology, Immunopharmacology and Treatment* (New York: Academic Press, 1973).

Austen, K. F., and Lichtenstein, L. M. (eds.): *Asthma: Physiology, Immunopharmacology and Treatment* (New York: Academic Press, 1973).

Austen, K. F., and Orange, R. P.: Bronchial asthma: The possible role of the chemical mediators of immediate hypersensitivity in the pathogenesis of subacute chronic disease, Am. Rev. Respir. Dis. 112:423, 1975.

Aviado, D. M. (ed.): *Krantz and Carr's Pharmacologic Principles of Medical Practice* (8th ed.; Baltimore: Williams & Wilkins Co., 1972).

Bouhuys, A.: Pulmonary response to bronchodilators, Am. Rev. Respir. Dis. (suppl.) 110:119, 1974.

Cropp, G. J. A.: The role of the parasympathetic nervous system in the maintenance of chronic airway obstruction in asthmatic children, Am. Rev. Respir. Dis. 112:599, 1975.

Fleish, J. H., Kent, K. M., and Cooper, T.: Drug Receptors in Smooth Muscle, in Austen, K. F., and Lichtenstein, L. M. (eds.): *Asthma: Physiolgy, Immunopharmacology and Treatment* (New York: Academic Press, 1973).

Gaddie, J., et al.: The effect of alpha adrenergic receptor-blocking drug on histamine sensitivity in bronchial asthma, Br. J. Dis. Chest 66:141, 1972.

Goodman, L. S., and Gilman, A.: *The Pharmacological Basis of Therapeutics* (5th ed.; New York: Macmillan Publishing Co., Inc., 1975).

Gross, G. N., Souhadra, J. F., and Farr, R. S.: The long term treatment of an asthmatic patient using phentolamine, Chest 66:397, 1974.

Hardman, J. G., et al.: the formation and metabolism of cyclic GMP, Ann. N.Y. Acad. Sci. 185:27, 1971.

Kalimer, M., Orange, R. P., and Austen, K. F.: Immunological release of histamine and slow-reacting substance of anaphylaxis in lung. IV. Enhancement of cholinergic and alpha adrenergic stimulation, J. Exp. Med. 136:556, 1972.

Kolata, G. B.: Cyclic GMP: Cellular regulatory agent? Science 182:149, 1973.

Lands, A. M. et al.: Differentiation of receptor systems activated by sympathomimetic amines, Nature 214:597, 1967.

Lichtenstein, L. M., and Margolis, S.: Histamine release *in vitro:* Inhibition by catecholamines and methylxanthines, Science 161:902, 1968.

Logsdon, P. J., et al.: The effect of phentolamine on adenylate cyclase and on isoproterenol stimulation in leukocytes from asthmatic and nonasthmatic subjects, J. Allergy Clin. Immunol. 52:148, 1973.

Middleton, E., Jr.: The biochemical basis for the modulation of allergic reactions by drugs, Pediatr. Clin. North Am. 22:111, 1975.

Murad, F.: Mechanism of action on some bronchodilators, Am. Rev. Respir. Dis. 110:111 (suppl.), 1974.

Nelson, H. S.: The beta adrenergic theory of bronchial asthma, Pediatr. Clin. North Am. 22:53, 1975.

Parker, C. D., Bilbo, R. E., and Reed, C. E.: Methacholine aerosol as test for bronchial asthma, Arch. Intern. Med. 115:452, 1965.

Patel, K. R., and Kerr, J. W.: The airways response to phenylephrine after blockade of alpha and beta receptors in extrinsic bronchial asthma, Clin. Allergy 3:439, 1973.

Rau, J. L.: Autonomic airway pharmacology, Respir. Care 22:263, 1977.

Reed, C. E.: The pathogenesis of asthma, Med. Clin. North Am. 58:55, 1974.

Said, S. I.: The lung in relation to vasoactive hormones, Fed. Proc. 32:1972, 1973.

Simonsson, B. G., et al.: *In vivo* and *in vitro* studies on α-receptors in human airways, Scand. J. Respir. Dis. 53:227, 1972.

Szentivanyi, A.: The beta adrenergic theory of the atopic abnormality in bronchial asthma, J. Allergy 42:203, 1968.

Yu, D. Y. C., Galant, S. P., and Gold, W. M.: Inhibition of antigen-induced bronchoconstriction by atropine in asthmatic subjects, J. Appl. Physiol. 32:823, 1972.

CHAPTER 4

# Sympathomimetic Bronchodilators

SYMPATHOMIMETIC BRONCHODILATORS comprise one of the most useful and potent groups of respiratory therapy drugs, and this class contains more specific drug agents than any other single class.

The direction of development for this class of drugs is *from* drugs activating both alpha *and* beta sites *to* very specific beta-two stimulants, giving bronchodilation with minimal or no cardiovascular and central nervous effects.

This orientation of drug research is best seen in a review of the chemical structures currently available or projected for the sympathomimetic class. In general, the trend has been from the catecholamines through resorcinols to saligenins. This is best illustrated through definitions and examples.

In Figure 4–1, the basic catecholamine structure is seen to be composed of a benzene ring with hydroxyl groups at the third and fourth carbon sites, and an amine side chain attached at the first carbon position.

*Catecholamine:* one of a group of similar compounds having a sympathomimetic action, the aromatic portion of whose molecule is catechol, and the diphatic portion an amine.

Examples of catecholamines are dopamine, epinephrine, norepinephrine, and isoproterenol. The first three occur naturally in the body, and there is evidence that an agent similar to isoproterenol may be found in the body. Catecholamines, or sympathomimetic amines, mimic the actions of epinephrine more or less precisely. In Figure 4–2, the basic catechol nucleus and the structural similarities of norepinephrine, epinephrine, and isoproterenol are shown. The relative degree of stimulation of alpha, beta-one, and beta-two receptors is indicated. Modifications to the side chain, such as with isoproterenol or isoetharine (Dilabron), increases the specificity of beta-one, and beta-two, respectively.

49

Catecholamines  { benzene ring
2 hydroxyl groups
amine side chain

Structure:

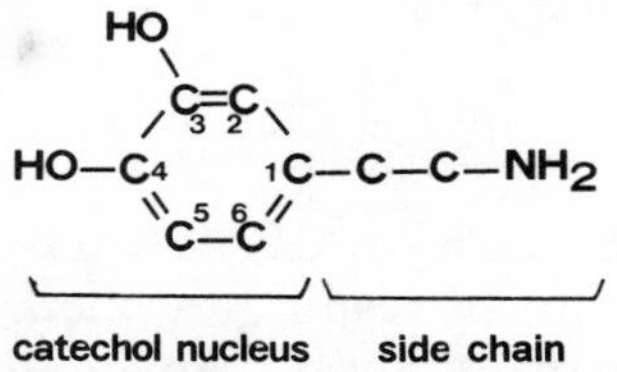

**Fig 4-1.**—The basic catecholamine structure showing the *catechol nucleus* (benzene ring and two hydroxyl groups) connected to the amine *side chain*.

Epinephrine substitutes a methyl group for a hydrogen attached to the side chain of norepinephrine, making the former an equal activator of alpha and beta receptors. As the bulk of the substitution on the side chain increases, the beta stimulation is increased and alpha activation is lessened. Isoproterenol is the best example of this, with strong beta stimulation and very little alpha stimulation. Isoetharine (Dilabron) adds an ethyl group to the amine side chain (see Fig 4–2), modifying the structure of isoproterenol and producing beta-two activity. Actually, bronchodilator activity is reduced by an approximate factor of 10 compared with isoproterenol, but cardiovascular stimulation is less by a factor of 300.

Following the introduction of isoetharine, an ingredient in Bronkosol, with its promise of preferential beta-two activity, research continued to find even more specific beta-two agents.

The catechol nucleus was modified by transferring the site of the hydroxyl radical at carbon-4 to carbon-5, producing a resorcinol nucleus seen in metaproterenol (Alupent, Metaprel) or terbutaline (Bricanyl), and greater beta-two specificity (Fig 4–3). Because of this modification of the catechol nucleus, the enzymes which inactivate isoproterenol do not affect metaproterenol. This gives metaproterenol a longer duration of activity. The changes seen in the structure of terbutaline (see Fig 4–3) produce bronchodilator activity twice as powerful as metaproterenol, with less cardiac stimulation.

Finally, further modification of the catechol nucleus yields salbutamol (albuterol), a beta-two sympathomimetic currently being reviewed for general use in the United States (Fig 4–4).

**CATECHOLAMINES IN RESPIRATORY THERAPY**

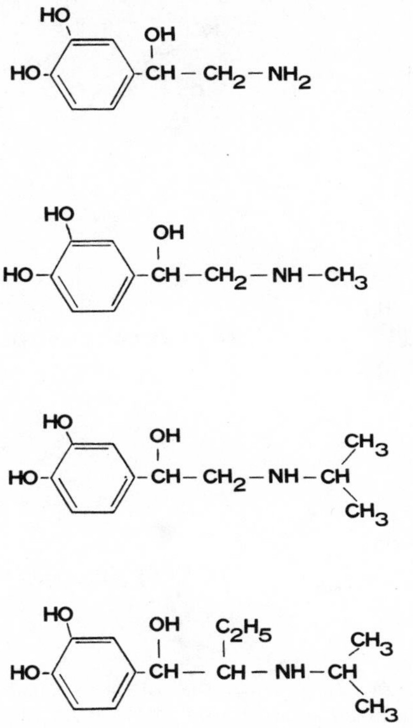

Norepinephrine ($\alpha > \beta$)

Epinephrine ($\alpha = \beta$)

Isoproterenol ($\alpha < \beta$)

Isoetharine ($\beta_2 > \beta_1$)

**Fig 4–2.**—Structural formulas for *norepinephrine, epinephrine, isoproterenol,* and *isoetharine.* The direction of activity is toward a specific beta-two stimulation.

The preceding review of the chemical structures seen with sympathomimetics is evidence of the very minor structural changes that can lead to very helpful changes in the physiologic effects of a drug. Most of this work of drug development is done synthetically in the laboratory, in contrast to other drug sources such as plants or animals.

## SPECIFIC SYMPATHOMIMETIC BRONCHODILATORS

### Epinephrine HCl

IDENTIFICATION: a catecholamine, a natural product of the adrenal medulla in man.

## ANALOGUES OF ISOPROTERENOL

Catechol nucleus ➔ Resorcinol nucleus

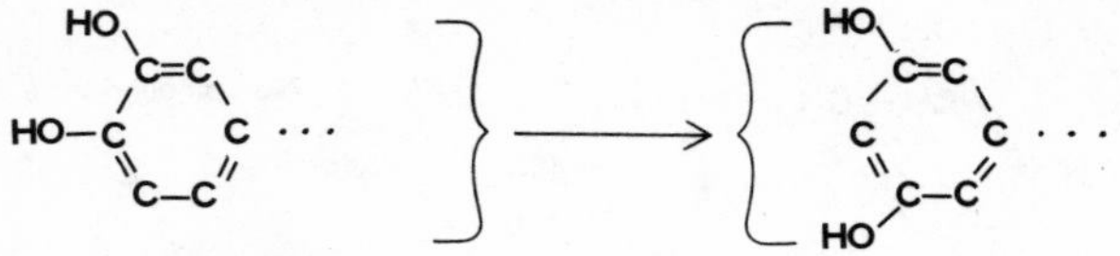

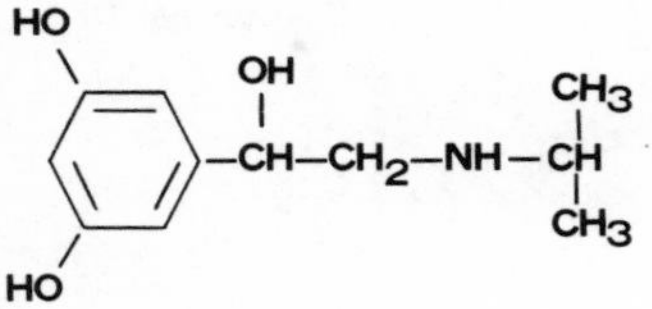

**Metaproterenol**

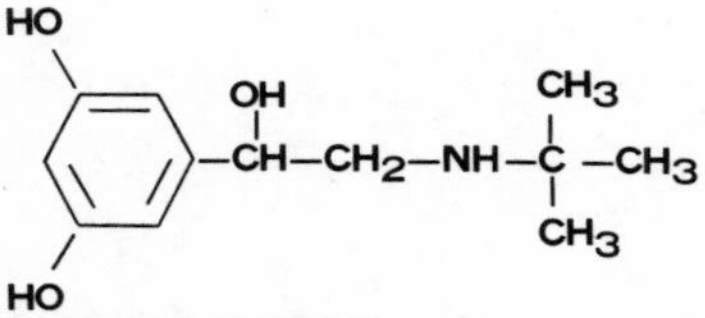

**Terbutaline**

**Fig 4–3.**—Modification of the benzene ring attachments produces the resorcinol nucleus seen in the beta-two stimulants, *metaproterenol* sulfate and *terbutaline* sulfate.

STRENGTH: 1:100 (1%, 10 mg/ml).

DOSAGE: 0.25–0.5 ml in 3–5 ml saline, by aerosol.

MODE OF ACTION: Epinephrine equally stimulates alpha and beta receptors to relax bronchial smooth muscle, shrink vasculature in the mucous membrane of the respiratory tract, and, unfortunately, increase the heart rate and force.

HAZARDS: tachycardia, increased blood pressure, and possibly mydriasis.

NOTES: epinephrine is metabolized by the enzyme catechol-*O*-methyltransferase to an inactive form, usually metanephrine.

$$\text{epinephrine} \xrightarrow{\text{COMT}} \text{metanephrine}$$

Catecholamines are also metabolized into inert adrenochromes by light, heat, or air. This is usually indicated by a pink or pinkish brown

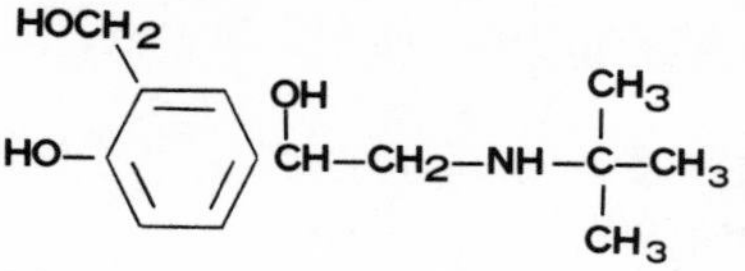

**Salbutamol**

**Fig 4–4.**—Additional modifications show production of a saligenin, such as *salbutamol*, with beta-two specific effects.

tinge in the solution. These adrenochromes are nontoxic, but there is some possibility that they may act as beta blockers. It is for this reason that most catecholamines such as epinephrine, racemic epinephrine, and other drugs such as isoetharine or isoproterenol are stored in dark-colored, amber bottles.

$$\text{catecholamines} \xrightarrow[\substack{\text{light} \\ \text{or} \\ \text{heat} \\ \text{or} \\ \text{air}}]{} \text{inert adrenochromes}$$

### Racemic epinephrine (Micronefrin, Vaponefrin)

IDENTIFICATION: a synthetic form of epinephrine.

STRENGTH: 2.25% (22.5 mg/ml).

DOSAGE: 0.25–0.5 ml in 3–5 ml normal saline.

MODE OF ACTION: The mode of action of racemic epinephrine is the same as with natural epinephrine, giving both alpha and beta stimulation. However, there is approximately one-half the vasopressor effect of natural epinephrine, because the racemic mixture is composed of two stereoisomers. The body normally manufactures mainly *l*-epinephrine, which is one of the stereoisomers and which is the only active form of epinephrine physiologically. The synthetic mixture is comprised of 50% *d*-epinephrine and 50% *l*-epinephrine. The *d*-epinephrine is inactive. Thus the result is a 50% diluted solution in terms of physiologic effect. The presence of the stereoisomers is indicated by the optical inactivity of the mixture since a stereoisomer is identified by its ability to polarize light; racemic epinephrine is optically inactive because the two stereoisomers are mutually cancelling. The concept of stereoisomers can be illustrated with a simple chemical structure (Fig 4–5).

HAZARDS: Racemic epinephrine has the same hazards as well as the same metabolism as natural epinephrine, simply with reduced effects.

## CONCEPT OF STEREOISOMERS

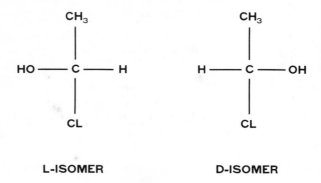

L-ISOMER                    D-ISOMER

__RACEMIC EPINEPHRINE__ - SYNTHETIC MIXTURE OF
L- AND D- EPINEPHRINE.  ONLY L-EPINEPHRINE
(NATURAL CATECHOLAMINE) IS PHYSIOLOGICALLY
ACTIVE.

**Fig 4–5.**—Simple representation of left- and right-handed stereoisomers.

### Isoproterenol (Isuprel)

IDENTIFICATION: a catecholamine.

STRENGTH: 1:200 (0.5%, 5 mg/ml).

DOSAGE: 0.25–0.5 ml in 3–5 ml normal saline, by aerosol.

MODE OF ACTION: Isoproterenol is one of the most pure beta stimulants, giving powerful beta-one and beta-two activation. This results in bronchial smooth muscle relaxation, pulmonary vasodilation, and also cardiac excitation.

HAZARDS: tachycardia, hypertension (initially).

NOTES: Isoproterenol has a 10–20 minute duration. It is metabolized by COMT as seen in the following scheme:

$$\text{isoproterenol} \xrightarrow{\text{COMT}} \text{3-methoxyisoproterenol}$$
(beta blocker, weak)

Interestingly enough, isoproterenol is metabolized to a weak beta blocker, and some have speculated that this is the cause of tachyphylaxis, or resistance to the drug's effects. When orally administered, the drug is very weak in its effects, because it is

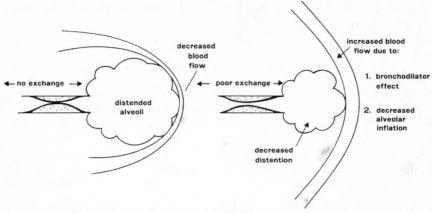

**Fig 4–6.**—Representation of hyperinflated, underperfused alveoli; isoproterenol is thought to increase blood flow and decrease alveolar distention, but without good alveolar exchange of inhaled gases. Venous admixture can result.

additionally inactivated in the gut and liver by conversion to a sulfate:

$$\text{oral drug} \xrightarrow[\text{sulfatase}]{\text{COMT}} \begin{cases} \text{3-methoxyisoproterenol} \\ \text{sulfate} \end{cases}$$

A *fall in $Pa_{O_2}$* has been noted with isoproterenol administration during asthmatic bronchospasm, as the ventilation improves and the attack is relieved. The mechanism for this seems to be an increase in perfusion of poorly ventilated portions of the lung (Fig 4–6). Isoproterenol could have two effects that cause this result:

1. Pulmonary vasodilation and increase in perfusion throughout the lung, which would unfortunately include underventilated alveoli.
2. Relief of hyperinflated (air-trapping) alveoli to decrease the overdistention. However, the decreased bronchospasm due to the isoproterenol may only allow the trapped air to escape, without immediately promoting good *exchange* of air. The $\dot{V}/\dot{Q}$ ratio will remain very low in these units, and can fall lower as relief of distention decreases vascular resistance, and as the drug increases vasodilation.

Such a view is compatible with the fact that an aerosol delivery of isoproterenol would preferentially be distributed to the better ventilated portions of the lungs initially.

## Isoproterenol and cyclopentamine (Aerolone)

IDENTIFICATION: This is a compound drug, consisting of an alpha (cyclopentamine) and a beta (isoproterenol) stimulant.

STRENGTH: cyclopentamine, 0.5% (5 mg/ml); isoproterenol, 0.25% (2.5 mg/ml).

DOSAGE: 0.5 ml in 3–5 ml of diluent.

MODE OF ACTION: Cyclopentamine, like phenylephrine, is a very pure alpha stimulant, and causes shrinkage of the mucous membrane. This is a decongestant effect similar to that obtained with phenylephrine. This decongestant effect is added to the strong beta action of isoproterenol which results therefore in both shrinking swollen membranes and relaxing constricted bronchial smooth muscle, to give an overall improvement of ventilation.

## Isoetharine (Bronkosol)

IDENTIFICATION: Isoetharine is a preferential beta-two stimulant formerly compounded with the strong alpha-stimulant phenylephrine. Isoetharine has a basic catecholamine structure, with an alpha-ethyl group added to the amine side chain.

STRENGTH: isoetharine (Dilabron), 1.0% (10 mg/ml).

DOSAGE: 0.25–0.5 ml in 3–5 ml saline.

MODE OF ACTION: Isoetharine is a primary beta-two stimulant to give bronchodilation with minimal cardiac side effects. Phenylephrine provided strong alpha stimulation to shrink congested membranes. This compound action was similar to that obtained with the isoproterenol-cyclopentamine combination (Aerolone). A third ingredient, thenyldiamine (an antihistamine) has been deleted for lack of evidence of efficacy. Isoetharine has $1/64$ to $1/16$ the strength of isoproterenol on bronchial smooth muscle, with a slower onset and longer duration of action, although the unmodified catechol nucleus is vulnerable to metabolism by COMT. However, isoetharine also has 300 times less effect on the cardiovascular system.

HAZARDS: Despite the beta-two action of the drug, the normal side effects of tachycardia and increase in blood pressure should be monitored, as with any sympathomimetic drug.

NOTE: As with the other sympathomimetic catecholamines, the drug is stored in dark bottles to prevent oxidation. If it is pinkish or discolored it should not be used. A pink tinge may be noticed in patient tubing or in the patient's secretions following nebulization therapy, because of the adrenochrome formation after treatment.

## Metaproterenol sulfate (Alupent, Metaprel, orciprenaline)

IDENTIFICATION: This is an analogue of isoproterenol with a resorcinol nucleus replacing the catechol nucleus. The hydroxyl group is on the carbon-5 position of the benzene ring instead of the carbon-4 position.

STRENGTH: metered-dose inhaler with 225 mg; 20 mg tablets for oral dose.

DOSAGE: 2–3 metered inhalations; 20 mg tablet orally.

MODE OF ACTION: This analogue of isoproterenol is $1/10$ to $1/40$ as strong, and primarily a beta-two stimulator, giving bronchodilation with minimal cardiac excitation. The 20 mg oral dose in adults gives bronchodilator effect which peaks in 1–2 hours, lasting for up to 4 hours. Inhaled doses of up to 1.5 mg give prompt bronchodilation without side effects. Metaproterenol is not metabolized by COMT, which accounts for the longer-acting duration than with isoproterenol. It is excreted as glucuronic acid conjugates.

HAZARDS: Although less likely than with other sympathomimetics which are not beta-two stimulants, tachycardia or hypertension may be seen.

CONTRAINDICATIONS: Metaproterenol should not be used with other sympathomimetics, because of possible additive and/or toxic effects, by patients with congestive heart failure. The drug should not be used during pregnancy or lactation or by women of childbearing age, unless the benefits outweigh the potential risks. Currently, metaproterenol is not approved for use by children under 12.

NOTE: This drug may or may not be directly administered by respiratory care personnel, but may be used by many patients receiving respiratory care through self-administered mistometers, or as a medication to be taken at home that is prescribed by the patient's attending physician.

## Terbutaline sulfate (Bricanyl, Brethine)

IDENTIFICATION: another analogue of isoproterenol, containing a resorcinol nucleus in place of the catechol nucleus.

STRENGTH: 0.1% (1 mg/ml ampule).

DOSAGE: 0.25 mg, subcutaneously; 5 mg tablets, orally.

MODE OF ACTION: This is a preferential beta-two stimulant, which is twice as potent as metaproterenol on bronchial smooth muscle, while giving less stimulation to cardiac muscle. The drug is relatively long-acting (3–5 hours), with minimal beta-one side effects. Unlike isoproterenol, it is *not* metabolized by COMT to a weak beta blocker such as 3-methoxyisoproterenol. The drug is effective given by mouth.

HAZARDS: Because of the beta-two preference of the drug, there is less likelihood of cardiovascular side effects; however these should always be monitored.

NOTE: As with metaproterenol, terbutaline may not be given directly by respiratory care personnel. This drug, however, represents an important step in the direction of development of beta-two bronchodilators.

## Salbutamol (albuterol)

IDENTIFICATION: This drug is a saligenin—not a catecholamine. It has not yet been approved for general use in the United States.

STRENGTH: not yet marketed in U.S.A.

DOSAGE: 100–200 μg by aerosol (0.1–0.2 mg) in .trial use; 2–5 mg orally.

MODE OF ACTION: Salbutamol is a selective beta-two stimulant, which is longer acting than isoproterenol (up to 6 hours duration). The effect of the drug may be longer acting after inhalation than after oral administration, because of the increased rate of absorption from the intestinal tract and rapid excretion in urine; there is slower absorption after inhalation. In test animals, the drug seems to be about $\frac{1}{5}$ as active as isoproterenol in preventing contraction of bronchial smooth muscle. There is virtually no alpha activity of the drug, and the least amount of beta-one activity is noted in comparison with any other beta-two stimulant.

### SUMMARY OF DRUG DEVELOPMENT IN SYMPATHOMIMETICS

The trend of development among sympathomimetic bronchodilators has been away from nonspecific beta stimulants toward specific beta-two stimulants with minimal beta-one effects. In general, there are several advantages seen with the newer beta-two stimulants:

1. There is the preferential beta-two activity;

2. There is no drop in $Pa_{O_2}$ caused by increased perfusion of underventilated lung seen with the catecholamines;
3. There is minimal central nervous system side effect (tremors, etc.);
4. There is prolonged action, since most are not metabolized by COMT;
5. The beta-two stimulants are not metabolized to beta blockers (such as occurs with isoproterenol).

## PROBLEMS WITH MISTOMETER DELIVERY SYSTEMS

The self-administered aerosol from a gas- or hand-powered cartridge nebulizer can pose serious problems, some of which are overlapping, such as the environmental effects and adverse patient reactions caused by these propellants. In more detail, the following possibilities must be considered with the mistometer type of bronchodilators:

1. There is some danger in permitting a patient to determine his own dosage of potent bronchodilator agents. Frightening bronchospasm can lead to abuse and psychological dependence.
2. Environmental effects of fluorocarbon propellants. In many cartridges, the aerosol is powered by supposedly inert fluorocarbons. Essentially, it is hypothesized, with some verifying evidence, that fluorocarbons are too inert to be chemically transformed, or absorbed by water, snow, or ice; they diffuse slowly aloft where, at 20–25 kilometers' altitude, ultraviolet radiation dissociates chlorine atoms. Chlorine can catalyze the breakdown of ozone into diatomic oxygen. The ozone acts as a protective layer to absorb ultraviolet radiation, shielding the surface of the earth. Loss of ozone depletes this layer. The exact consequences are difficult to predict, but may involve increases in skin cancer.
3. The locked-lung syndrome. In the 1960s, asthma mortality among users of hand nebulizers in England and Wales jumped significantly. Overuse of the cartridges at the expense of alternate, superior therapy appears to be implicated, through one or more of the following mechanisms:
   a. Beta blockade brought about through accumulated levels of the beta-blocking metabolite of isoproterenol, 3-methoxyisoproterenol. Many argue this metabolite is too weak to result in irreversible bronchospasm. There is evidence that prolonged use of isoproterenol causes diminished response to sympathomimetics.

b. Altered $\dot{V}/\dot{Q}$ ratios, with pulmonary vasodilation in under-ventilated areas of the lung, all leading to decreased $Pa_{O_2}$ and hypoxemia. Isoproterenol by aerosol promotes bronchodilation in the well-ventilated portions of the lung, while pulmonary blood flow increases to poorly ventilated areas, giving venous admixture.

c. There may be cardiotoxicity of the propellants. The "inert" fluorocarbons can cause arrhythmias in high serum concentrations.

d. All of the preceding, especially a and b, may have been at fault because the English inhalers delivered approximately 5 times the dosage strength of American mistometers, where such an outbreak of death has not occurred.

## REFERENCES

Avner, S. E.: β-Adrenergic bronchodilators, Pediatr. Clin. North Am. 22:129, 1975.

Bierman, C. W., and Pierson, W. E.: Hand nebulizers and asthma therapy in children and adolescents, Pediatrics 54:668, 1974.

Chick, T. W., et al.: Effects of bronchodilators on the distribution of ventilation and perfusion in asthma, Chest (suppl.) 63:11S, 1973.

Connolly, M. E., et al.: Acquired resistance to beta stimulants—a possible explanation for the rise in the asthma death rate in Britain, Chest, 63:165, 1973.

Dulfano, M. J.: The new oral bronchodilators, Chest 68:133, 1975.

Dulfano, M. J., and Glass, P.: Evaluation of a new β2 adrenergic receptor stimulant, terbutaline, in bronchial asthma: Oral comparison with ephedrine, Curr. Ther. Res. 15:150, 1973.

Frank, R.: Are aerosol sprays hazardous? (editorial), Am. Rev. Respir. Dis. 112:485, 1975.

Middleton, E., Jr., and Finke, S. R.: Metabolic response to epinephrine in bronchial asthma, J. Allergy 42:288, 1968.

Murray, A. B., et al.: The effects of pressurized isoproterenol and salbutamol in asthmatic children, Pediatrics 54:746, 1974.

Sobol, B. J., et al.: The response to isoproterenol in normal subjects and subjects with asthma, Am. Rev. Respir. Dis. 109:290, 1974.

Stolley, P. D.: Asthma mortality: A possible explanation of international variations, Chest (suppl.) 63:18S, 1973.

# CHAPTER 5

# Parasympatholytic and Xanthine Bronchodilators

TWO OTHER CLASSES OF DRUGS which are able to provide bronchodilator action are parasympatholytics, such as atropine, and xanthines, such as aminophylline.

The basic mode of action of each of these can be quickly understood in terms of the cyclic AMP–cyclic GMP schema discussed earlier when outlining the autonomic nervous system (see Chapter 3). That schema is given in Figure 5–1.

If, as research indicates, smooth muscle relaxation and contraction is mediated through the intracellular nucleotides cyclic AMP and cyclic GMP, then any class of drugs which affects these nucleotides could produce changes in smooth muscle tone. Specifically, beta sympathomimetics have been seen to increase cyclic AMP through interaction with the receptor enzyme, adenyl cyclase (Chapter 4). This results in the relaxation of smooth muscle in bronchioles or blood vessels. Conversely, a beta blocker, such as propranolol (Inderal), might decrease cyclic AMP, causing contraction of the smooth muscle. Cyclic AMP concentrations in the cell could also be increased in two further ways: by blocking, or inhibiting, the enzyme phosphodiesterase which inactivates cyclic AMP; and by decreasing the production of cyclic GMP. Xanthines operate to inhibit phosphodiesterase, and although there is no increased *production* of cyclic AMP, the overall concentration builds because of slower inactivation of the substance. Parasympatholytics can serve to block parasympathetic-induced cyclic GMP. Cyclic GMP produces an effect opposite to that of cyclic AMP, which is contraction of smooth muscle. Thus a parasympathomimetic such as methacholine can "challenge" hyperreactive airways to cause bronchoconstriction. Normal sympathetic and parasympathetic innervation are thought to produce a balance of cyclic AMP and GMP, i.e., neither constriction nor relaxation. Therefore, if cyclic GMP is *de-*

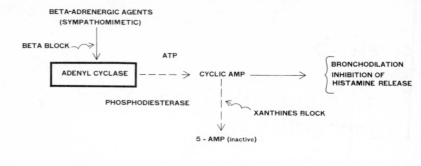

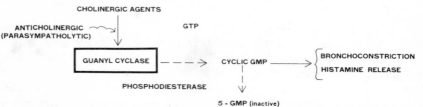

**Fig 5–1.**—Schema of sympathetic (adrenergic) and parasympathetic (cholinergic) nucleotide mediators.

*creased,* through parasympathetic block, the net effect is a *relative increase* in cyclic AMP. In other words, there is less cyclic GMP to oppose the relaxing effect of cyclic AMP, and the relaxation becomes predominant. Physiologically this is bronchodilation.

## PARASYMPATHOLYTIC AGENTS

As a classic parasympatholytic, atropine blocks parasympathetic-induced glandular secretion, to dry up nasal, lacrimal, and bronchial glands. Secretions, particularly mucus, can become thick, and the mouth dry. Mucus plugging of small airways is considered a hazardous side effect. The major therapeutic effect causing renewed interest in atropine and its derivatives is the block in cyclic GMP, giving a relative increase in cyclic AMP and promoting bronchodilation. Not only is atropine able to decrease bronchospasm due to irritants (dust, pollen, aerosols, exercise) but also that due to antigen-induced histamine release of allergic asthma, which is enhanced by cyclic GMP. Interestingly, the term *belladonna* (which means "beautiful lady") was used for the plant from which atropine is extracted because of the practice of Italian ladies who ingested the plant to dilate their pupils, thereby enhancing their beauty.

## Atropine sulfate

IDENTIFICATION: Atropine (*dl*-hyoscyamine) is an extract of the night-
shade plant *Atropa belladonna,* a naturally occurring alkaloid. The
*l*-isomers are more potent in their effects on both the peripheral
and central nervous system.

STRENGTH: 0.2% to 1.0% solution for aerosol.

DOSAGE: 3–5 ml for nebulization.

MODE OF ACTION: competitive inhibition with acetylcholine for
receptor sites on postsynaptic membranes. It is thought to block
the activation of cyclic GMP to prevent bronchospasm due to
irritation of vagal epithelial receptors in trachea and bronchi, or
due to antigen-antibody reactions in the lung. Pretreatment with
IV atropine has prevented bronchospasm when asthmatics were
challenge-tested with methacholine (parasympathomimetic) or
with inhaled antigens (in 8 of 20 patients, in one study). Atropine
by aerosol has also caused improvement of airway resistance and
forced expiratory flows in asthmatics with measurable airway
obstruction even between acute episodes. Since atropine or other
parasympatholytics are not direct smooth muscle relaxants, but
can only block parasympathetic-induced bronchial tone and tight-
ness, it is indicated that some reversible airway obstruction is
mediated by parasympathetic impulse.

HAZARDS: thickening of bronchial secretions, mucus plugging, increase in heart rate.

NOTES: Atropine has traditionally been used as a preoperative drying
agent for secretions or as an agent to combat bradycardia by
blocking vagal (parasympathetic) inhibition of heart rate. Now
atropine is being used as a bronchodilator.


## Aerosol Sch 1000 (ipratropium bromide)

IDENTIFICATION: a derivative of atropine, a tropic acid ester with an
isopropyl group on the nitrogen atom, currently being tested for
use as a bronchodilator.

STRENGTH: (experimentally) 40–80 µg.

DOSAGE: single metered-dose inhaler.

MODE OF ACTION: relief of bronchospasm, probably through its
parasympatholytic effect in blocking cyclic GMP. The drug produces bronchodilation 5 minutes after administration by aerosol,
has a duration of 4 hours, with no known atropine-like side effects,
or other side effects. The major site of action appears to be in large

airways. The lack of side effects, especially thickened secretions, makes this drug of great potential for therapeutic use in airway obstruction which proves to be partially or completely mediated by the parasympathetic nervous system.

## XANTHINE AGENTS

Xanthines are related chemically to the natural metabolite xanthine, which is a precursor of uric acid.

The three xanthines used therapeutically are:

Caffeine—found in the seeds of the coffee plant.

Theobromine—found in the seeds of the cacao (chocolate) plant.

Theophylline—found in tea leaves.

All xanthines have the following effects:

1. Cerebral stimulant
2. Skeletal muscle stimulant
3. Bronchodilator
4. Pulmonary vasodilator
5. Smooth muscle relaxant
6. Coronary vasodilator
7. Cardiac stimulant
8. Diuretic

Each xanthine, however, differs in the degree of response elicited for given effects. Theophylline is most intense in effects 3 through 8, and is therefore preferred for bronchodilation, pulmonary vasodilation, and, in general, for smooth muscle relaxation.

Although respiratory care personnel will probably not directly administer xanthines, this group offers a primary method of attacking bronchospasm and asthma.

*Prophylactically,* theophylline (aminophylline) is administered *orally* to those with chronic asthma, or impending attacks. Theophylline is given in several forms and mixtures besides aminophylline. Theophylline has been combined with potassium iodide (an expectorant promoting mucus production), with ephedrine (sympathomimetic), with glyceryl guaiacolate (an emollient with possible mucolytic and expectorant effects), and with alcohol. A more recent name for glyceryl guaiacolate is guaifenesin. Several of these agents and compounds are listed next, with dosage strengths and forms indicated.

Therapeutically, aminophylline, given IV in large doses, is a key maneuver in treating status asthmaticus, and is used with epinephrine subcutaneously, and oxygen therapy initially. The basic effects on the lung are:

1. Decreased airway resistance (bronchodilation)
2. Decreased pulmonary vascular resistance (vasodilation)
3. Stimulated ventilation

### Theophylline ethylenediamine (aminophylline)

IDENTIFICATION: Aminophylline is a double salt composed of theophylline and ethylenediamine, which increases the aqueous solubility of theophylline to permit IV administration of large doses (250–500 mg) of aminophylline.

STRENGTH: 0.25 gm in 20 ml or 0.5 gm in 40 ml of solution; 0.2 gm per tablet.

DOSAGE: 0.25 gm or 0.5 gm given intravenously over 20 to 40 minutes, or 0.4 gm orally (2 tablets).

MODE OF ACTION: Aminophylline also operates within the cyclic AMP system, but instead of directly stimulating the beta receptor, these xanthines inhibit the enzyme phosphodiesterase to block the breakdown of cyclic AMP to an inactive form. Xanthines do not equally inhibit phosphodiesterase enzymes which inactivate cyclic GMP, and therefore there is not a concomitant rise in cyclic GMP to oppose the relaxing effect of cyclic AMP on smooth muscle. The difficulty in regulating dosages of aminophylline may be related to an effect on more than one phosphodiesterase enzyme.

NOTE: Aminophylline has been given in a dosage of 0.25 gm in 1.0 ml (25% solution) of distilled water, by both hand-bulb nebulizer (using 6 inhalations) and oxygen-powered aerosol. The aerosol is usually irritating to the pharynx, has a bitter taste, and can cause coughing and wheezing. In asthmatic patients, there had been no significant improvement in vital capacity and no protection against challenge with aerosol or intravenous histamine and methacholine, which produced bronchospasm and dyspnea. Both oral and intravenous aminophylline have been demonstrated to provide protection against histamine or methacholine challenge tests.

### Theophylline capsules (Elixophyllin)

IDENTIFICATION: anhydrous theophylline in a suspension of polyethylene glycol.

STRENGTH: 200 mg per capsule.

DOSAGE: adults, 200 mg (1 capsule) 3 times daily.

## Theophylline elixir (Elixophyllin)

IDENTIFICATION: anhydrous theophylline in 20% alcohol.
STRENGTH: theophylline 80 mg/15 ml.
DOSAGE: maintenance dose, 30 ml 3 times daily.


## Ephedrine, theophylline, glyceryl guaiacolate, and phenobarbital (Bronkotabs)

IDENTIFICATION: a tablet consisting of the compounded ingredients just given.
STRENGTH: Each tablet contains ephedrine sulfate 24 mg; theophylline 100 mg; glyceryl guaiacolate 100 mg; phenobarbital 8 mg.
DOSAGE: 1 tablet 3–4 times daily.
MODE OF ACTION: As a compound, several actions are expected from various ingredients. Ephedrine provides alpha and beta stimulation, and theophylline inhibits phosphodiesterase. Together these ingredients produce increased levels of cyclic AMP, and bronchodilation. Glyceryl guaiacolate provides soothing effect on upper airways, particularly with irritating, nonproductive cough, and may lower mucus viscosity. Phenobarbital is intended to calm anxiety, to allow slower, more efficient ventilatory patterns.
NOTE: Normally, sedatives are never encouraged in patients with breathing difficulties, since such agents dull reflex sensitivity of chemoreceptors to $CO_2$, and may lead to hypoventilation, hypercapnea, and may worsen hypoxemia. For example, a patient in the emergency room in acute asthma would not be sedated since he/she needs to continue efforts to breathe.


## Theophylline and guaifenesin (Asbron G)

IDENTIFICATION: a compound containing theophylline sodium glycinate (xanthine) and guaifenesin (recent name for glyceryl guaiacolate).
STRENGTH: Each tablet contains theophylline sodium glycinate, 300 mg; guaifenesin, 100 mg. Each 15 ml of elixir, same.
DOSAGE: 1–2 tablets 3–4 times daily; 15–30 ml 3–4 times daily.
MODE OF ACTION: The xanthine provides bronchodilation while guaifenesin is an expectorant. Note the lack of the sympathomimetic component (ephedrine) or the sedative (phenobarbital).

REFERENCES

Chervinsky, P.: Double-blind study of ipratropium bromide, a new anticholinergic bronchodilator (abstract), J. Allergy Clin. Immunol. 57:261, 1976.

Cropp, G. J. A.: The role of the parasympathetic nervous system in the maintenance of chronic airway obstruction in asthmatic children, Am. Rev. Respir. Dis. 112:599, 1975.

Emergil, C., et al.: A new parasympatholytic bronchodilator: A study of its onset of effect after inhalation, Curr. Ther. Res. 17:215, 1975.

Etter, R. L., et al.: Effects of theophylline-alcohol with potassium iodide in asthmatic patients, Ann. Allergy 27:70, 1969.

Gayrard, P., et al.: Bronchoconstrictor effects of a deep inspiration in patients with asthma, Am. Rev. Respir. Dis. 111:433, 1975.

Gold, W. M.: Vagally-mediated reflex bronchoconstriction in allergic asthma, Chest (suppl.) 63:11S, 1973.

Harnett, J., and Spector, S. L.: Blocking effect of Sch 1000, isoproterenol, and the combination on methacholine and histamine inhalations (Abstract), J. Allergy Clin. Immunol. 57:261, 1976.

Jackson, R. H., et al.: Clinical evaluation of Elixophyllin (theophylline elixir) with correlation of pulmonary function studies and theophylline serum levels in acute and chronic asthmatic patients, Dis. Chest 45:75, 1964.

Jackson, R. H., et al.: Blood levels following oral administration of theophylline preparations, Ann. Allergy 31:413, 1973.

Jezek, V., et al.: The effect of aminophylline on the respiration and pulmonary circulation, Clin. Sci. 38:549, 1970.

Lichtenstein, L. M., and Margolis, S.: Histamine release in vitro: Inhibition by catecholamines and methylxanthines, Science 161:902, 1968.

Petrie, G. R., and Palmer, K. N. V.: Comparison of aerosol ipratropium bromide and salbutamol in chronic bronchitis and asthma, Br. Med. J. 1:430, 1975.

Richards, R. K.: Toxicity of theophylline-ephedrine-barbiturate mixtures, J. Pharmacol. Exp. Ther. 72:33, 1942.

Segal, M. S., et al.: Evaluation of therapeutic substances employed for the relief of bronchospasm. VI. Aminophylline, J. Clin. Invest. 28:1182, 1949.

Segal, M. S.: The Management of the Patient with Severe Bronchial Asthma (Springfield, Ill.: Charles C Thomas, 1950), pp. 49–51.

Segal, M. S.: Aminophylline: A clinical overview, Adv. Asthma Allergy 2:17, 1975.

Storms, W. W., DoPico, G. A., and Reed, C. E.: Aerosol Sch 1000, Am. Rev. Respir. Dis. 111:419, 1975.

Sutherland, E. W. and Rall, T. W.: The relation of adenosine-3[1], 5[1]-phosphate and phosphorylase to the action of catecholamines and other hormones, Pharmacol. Rev. 12:265, 1960.

Weinberger, M. M., and Bronsky, E. A.: Interaction of ephedrine and theophylline, Clin. Pharmacol. Ther. 17:585, 1975.

Yeager, H., et al.: Asthma: Comparative bronchodilator effects of ipratropium bromide and isoproterenol, J. Clin. Pharmacol. 16:198, 1976.

Yu, D. Y. C., Galant, S. P., and Gold, W. M.: Inhibition of antigen-induced bronchoconstriction by atropine in asthmatic subjects, J. Appl. Physiol. 32:823, 1972.

CHAPTER 6

# Mucolytics

IT was previously stated that the main purpose of respiratory therapy pharmacology is airway patency, accomplished through smooth muscle relaxation or control and reduction of pulmonary secretions. The sympathomimetics, parasympatholytics, and xanthines that have been considered have all resulted in relaxation of bronchial smooth muscle. Mucolytics are the first class of drugs to be considered that directly control pulmonary secretions.

## PHYSIOLOGY AND NATURE OF MUCUS

One of the major defense mechanisms of the lung is the self-renewing, self-cleansing mucociliary escalator. Mucus provides a blanket of normally sterile, somewhat sticky substance to trap debris and, in combination with the beating cilia, remove the debris toward the larynx, where the secretions and any debris can be expectorated or swallowed. The mucus blanket is a somewhat stratified substance, as can be seen in Figure 6–1. It is made up of basically two layers, with the gel being the outer, sticky layer; and the sol, the inner watery solution directly bathing the cilia. This blanket lines the inner surface of the conducting airways in the lung from at least the terminal bronchioles on up to the trachea and larynx. Within the watery sol, the cilia beat, moving the mucus blanket toward the glottis at approximately 2 centimeters per minute. The tracheobronchial tree of a normal adult produces approximately 100 ml per day of secretion. These secretions are produced by surface goblet cells and submucosal glands. Submucosal glands are generally of two types: serous (granular) cells; and mucous cells (see Fig 6–1). These glands are under parasympathetic (vagal) control.

Normal mucus has the following approximate composition:
95% water
2% glycoprotein—Mucus is a polypeptide with saccharide side
    chains. The presence of the side chains as well as the length of the

68

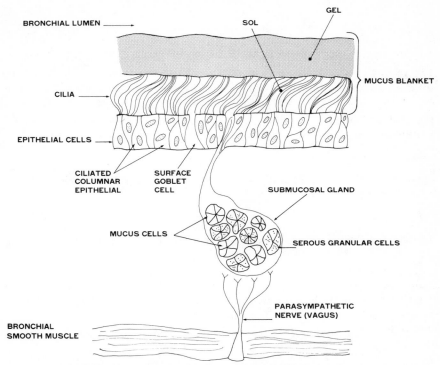

CROSS SECTION, BRONCHIOLE WALL

**Fig 6–1.**—Mucociliary mechanism in the lung.

polypeptides determines the *viscosity* of the mucus. This glycoprotein fibril network can be visualized by staining with toluidine
blue O.

1% carbohydrate

1% lipid

0.03% DNA—In infection the cellular bacterial debris which contains DNA increases radically. Deoxyribonucleoprotein fibrils
from disintegrated leukocytes become part of the gel structure,
increasing mucus tenacity. In this situation secretions are called
purulent, are frequently colored, and sometimes foul smelling.
Normal, uninfected mucus is colorless.

The term *sputum* is a more general term than mucus, and includes
mucus, nasal secretions, as well as salivary gland secretion. Sputum is
this mixed substance that is present in the oropharyngeal region.

Mucus viscosity can be decreased by any or all of the following
substances or mechanisms. Each action is related to the composition of
mucus.

1. Hydration—through normal saline or distilled water;
2. Increased pH levels in the tracheobronchial tree—accomplished through bicarbonate;
3. Proteolytic enzymes—pancreatic dornase;
4. Rupture of disulfide linkage—accomplished with acetylcysteine.

These basic actions have defined the agents most useful in reducing mucus viscosity. It is important to differentiate mucolytics from the class of drugs known as surface-active agents. Mucolytics have as a primary purpose a decrease in viscosity, whereas surface-active agents primarily attack the surface tension of the secretions.

## SPECIFIC MUCOLYTIC AGENTS

### Humidifiers

IDENTIFICATION: Three types of agents are used for their water content. The osmotic relationship of each of these agents to normal body fluid is:

normal saline—isotonic to body fluid

half-normal saline—hypotonic to body fluid

distilled water—hypotonic to body fluid

STRENGTH: normal saline (0.9%); half-normal saline (0.45%); distilled water.

DOSAGE: 3–5 ml for aerosol treatment, or by direct tracheal instillation of normal saline (0.9%). Each of the agents may be used as diluting agents for another active ingredient, or by themselves to provide humidification.

MODE OF ACTION: One of the best agents for reducing the viscosity of mucus is plain water since the primary constituent of mucus is 95% water. In application, this means that mucus needs a large amount of water to remain near its normal viscosity. Regardless of the cause of thickening, water is useful for returning mucus to its normal viscosity. Normal saline is used as isotonic solution to minimize tracheobronchial irritation. Distilled water, being hypotonic, is sometimes used deliberately, however, as an irritant to provoke sputum samples for a specimen. The lower osmolarity of plain water causes it to be absorbed by the hypertonic mucus, promoting expectoration. Half-normal saline is actually hypotonic to body fluid, but during aerosolization the saline may evaporate some of its water, raising its osmolarity much closer, or equal to, body fluid. In the same way, normal saline during evaporation under aerosolization may actually become hypertonic to body fluid.

NOTE: Bacteriostatic additives—When a vial of normal saline or distilled water is labeled bacteriostatic, preservatives have been added to the drug. Certain of these preservatives are parabens which are alkyl esters of parahydroxy-benzoic acid. These are of two types, either methylparabens or propylparabens. Parabens may sensitize the skin and induce allergic reactions such as mucous membrane irritation, or dermatitis. There is a low incidence of toxicity however. For aerosolization or other direct treatment of the tracheobronchial tree, such as during irrigation, physiologic saline or saline and distilled water without additives is preferred.

## Acetylcysteine (Mucomyst, Mucomyst-10)

IDENTIFICATION: This is an acetyl derivative of the amino acid cysteine.

STRENGTH: 10%, or 20% (100 mg/ml, 200 mg/ml).

DOSAGE: 2–3 ml undiluted.

MODE OF ACTION: Acetylcysteine breaks mucus chains by replacing the disulfide (SS) bond in mucus with its own sulfhydryl groups, as seen in Figure 6–2. Acetylcysteine does not attack the main protein chain. Replacing the disulfide bond weakens the structure, and this lowers the viscosity (see Fig 6–2). Optimal action is at 7.0–9.0 pH, as indicated in the graph seen in Figure 6–3. There is reduced mucolytic action in acidic pH.

HAZARDS: Acetylcysteine has induced bronchospasm, and many prefer to use a bronchodilator additive with the drug. This is especially useful if the 20% concentration is used. In addition, acetylcysteine is reactive with rubber, copper, iron, and cork. EDTA (ethylenediaminetetraacetic acid) is added to acetylcysteine as a chelating agent to tie up heavy metal ions. This preserves the activity of the drug, by preventing any deterioration through reaction with metal ions. Acetylcysteine is incompatible with the following antibiotics since it inhibits their antibacterial action:

> sodium ampicillin
> amphotericin B
> erythromycin
> tetracyclines

The rotten-egg odor of acetylcysteine that is due to the sulfhydryl

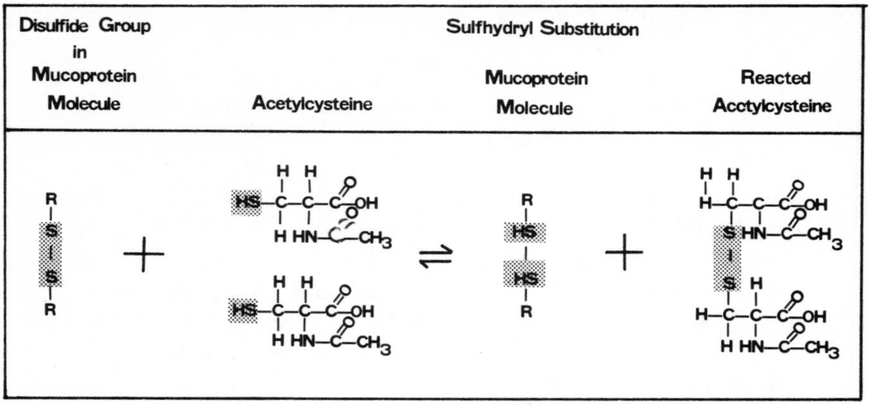

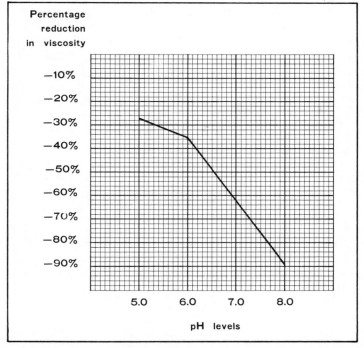

**Fig 6–2.**—Mechanism of action by which *acetylcysteine* reduces the viscosity of mucus. Acetylcysteine substitutes the sulfhydryl for the disulfide bonds. (From *Professional Handbook of Clinical Experience* [Evansville, Ind.: Mead-Johnson & Co., 1970]. Used by permission.)

**Fig 6–3.**—The relation of pH to the mucolytic activity of acetylcysteine. Optimal pH levels are between 7.0 and 9.0. (From *Professional Handbook of Clinical Experience* [Evansville, Ind.: Mead-Johnson & Co., 1970]. Used by permission.)

radicals can cause nausea in patients. This is a hazard to be watched for by the therapist or technician.

NOTE: Acetylcysteine is rapidly degraded to cysteine by the liver. Ciliary activity is not inhibited by the drug. Discard opened bottles after 96 hours. A slight purple color which is due to the EDTA combining with heavy metal ions does not affect the activity of the drug. The odor produced during nebulization is due to approximately one part per million of hydrogen sulfide emitted when the drug is degraded.

## Pancreatic dornase (Dornavac)

IDENTIFICATION: No longer available. A nonspecific proteolytic enzyme derived from beef; recently removed from the market by the FDA.

STRENGTH: 50,000 units/ml. The drug came as a powder containing 100,000 units, with a 2 ml vial of sterile diluent to reconstitute the powder.

DOSAGE: 50,000 to 100,000 units per treatment, 2–3 times daily.

MODE OF ACTION: This drug depolymerized DNA strands found in cellular debris associated with infected and purulent sputum. The drug was particularly useful when heavy infection of the pulmonary secretions was present. It has been suggested that dornase facilitated *topical* (local, not systemic) antibiotic therapy: depolymerization of the DNA prevents inactivation of antibiotics which can result from binding to DNA in the secretions. Thus, a mixture of dornase and a suitable antibiotic offered a potentially effective combination for dealing with infected mucus by helping the antibiotic to reach the source of infection.

HAZARDS: Since the drug was a nonspecific proteolytic enzyme it attacked any protein, not just the DNA of infected mucus. Pharyngeal soreness and irritation were sometimes noticed as side effects. It was recommended that patients gargle after treatment by aerosol, and that the drug be used for brief periods at a time (5–10 minutes) over not more than several days.

NOTE: The drug should be refrigerated. There is a decreasing potency after the drug is opened, and it should be discarded after one week following opening.

## Sodium bicarbonate

IDENTIFICATION: This is a weak base.

STRENGTH: 2% by aerosol (20 mg/ml). A commercially available unit-dose preparation has a 4.2% (42 mg/ml) strength.

DOSAGE: 2–5 ml for nebulization. For home use, 1 teaspoon baking soda in a cup of water.

MODE OF ACTION: Bicarbonate acts to increase the local bronchial pH, and thereby break the saccharide side chains in the mucus chain to decrease the mucus viscosity.

HAZARDS: Although the respiratory tract may reach a pH of 8.3 topically without damage, a too alkaline pH may result in bronchial mucosal irritation.

NOTE: It would take excessive amounts of bicarbonate by aerosolization to significantly affect systemic pH of the body.

## CLINICAL USE OF MUCOLYTICS

Use of humidifying agents to hydrate, and thereby liquefy, secretions by *aerosol* administration is probably ineffective because of the small amount of water actually contained in aerosols. Better forms of hydration are adequate oral intake of fluid, such as a glass of water or juice (*not* beer, tea, or cola, all of which have a diuretic effect). Humidifying agents, however, may be used with good results in each of the following cases:

1. To humidify dry inspired gases during IPPB or oxygen therapy;
2. As a diluent for other drug agents such as bronchodilators;
3. For sputum induction, where the preferred method of nebulization is by ultrasonic nebulizer to provide optimum particle size with larger amounts of the saline or water.

In brief, water by aerosol is not an effective mucolytic, but water through oral intake is the best chronic regulator of mucus viscosity.

Both dornase and acetylcysteine have been shown objectively through viscosity measurements to be effective in thinning, or reducing, the viscosity of secretions. A third proteolytic enzyme, trypsin, has also been demonstrated as effective. The drug of choice with thick, tenacious secretions, however, is acetylcysteine—and direct, liquid instillation is more effective than aerosol administration. Prompt suctioning may be necessary to remove the massive liquefaction of the secretions.

The proteolytic enzymes (dornase, trypsin) are irritants to respiratory mucosa through their nonspecific proteolytic action. They may represent an additional hazard as potential antigenic stimulants, causing sensitization of patients. Finally, since proteases (proteolytic enzymes), and the lack of protease inhibitors such as alpha$_1$-antitrypsin, may be involved in the pathogenesis of emphysema, it is concluded that aerosolized dornase or trypsin is not well indicated from what is known presently.

The use of mucolytics does not register improvement in spirometric values such as FEV, FVC, MVV, $FEF_{2-12}$, or $FEF_{25-75}$. Subjective feelings of improvement are related to addition of a bronchodilator, not to the mucolytic. This does *not* indicate that mucolysis does not occur, which has been objectively verified by viscosity measurements, but rather that decreased viscosity favors expectoration/aspiration more than ventilatory flow rates.

For routine *maintenance* therapy of patients with chronically thick secretions, a planned program of adequate and appropriate fluid intake, bronchial hygiene, exercise, bronchodilator and antibiotic therapy—as needed—is preferential to chronic use of mucolytics.

## REFERENCES

Barton, A. D.: Aerosolized detergents and mucolytic agents in the treatment of stable chronic obstructive pulmonary disease, Am. Rev. Respir. Dis. 110:104, 1974.

Barton, A. D., and Lourenco, R. V.: Bronchial secretions and mucociliary clearance, Arch. Intern. Med. 131:140, 1973.

Barton, A. D., et al.: Biochemical characteristics affecting the consistency of bronchial secretions, Chest (suppl.) 63:59S, 1973.

Bernstein, L. I., and Ausdenmore, R. W.: Iatrogenic bronchospasm occurring during clinical trials of a new mucolytic agent, acetylcysteine, Dis. Chest 46:469, 1964.

Dippy, J. E., and Davis, S. S.: Rheological assessment of mucolytic agents on sputum of chronic bronchitics, Thorax 24:707, 1969.

Eriksson, S.: Studies in alpha-1-antitrypsin deficiency, Acta Med. Scand. (suppl.) 177:432, 1965.

Gibson, L. E.: Use of water vapor in the treatment of lower respiratory disease, Am. Rev. Respir. Dis. 110:100, 1974.

Kueppers, F., and Black, L. F.: Alpha-1 antitrypsin and its deficiency, Am. Rev. Respir. Dis. 110:176, 1974.

Lieberman, J.: Alpha₁-antitrypsin deficiency, Med. Clin. North Am. 57:691, 1973.

Lieberman, J.: The appropriate use of mucolytic agents, Am. J. Med. 49:1, 1970.

Lieberman, J.: Dornase aerosol effect on sputum viscosity in cases of cystic fibrosis, J.A.M.A. 205:114, 1968.

Mittman, C. (ed.): *Pulmonary Emphysema and Proteolysis* (New York: Academic Press, 1972).

Moser, K. M., and Rhodes, P. G.: Acute effects of aerosolized NAC upon spirometic measurements in subjects with and without obstructive pulmonary disease, Dis. Chest 40:37, 1966.

Rao, S., et al.: Acute effects of nebulization of N-acetylcysteine on pulmonary mechanics and gas exchange, Am. Rev. Respir. Dis. 102:17, 1970.

Reas, H. W.: The use of acetylcysteine in the treatment of cystic fibrosis, J. Pediatr. 65:542, 1964.

Sheffner, A. L., et al.: The in vitro reduction in viscosity of human tracheo-bronchial secretions by acetylcysteine, Am. Rev. Respir. Dis. 90:721, 1964.

Spier, R., Witebsky, E., and Paine, J. R.: Aerosolized pancreatic dornase and antibiotics in pulmonary infections: Use in patients with post-operative and non-operative infections, J.A.M.A. 178:878, 1961.

Unger, L., and Unger, A. H.: Trypsin inhalation in respiratory conditions associated with thick sputum: Its use in bronchiectasis, acute atelectasis, infectious bronchitis, bronchial asthma, emphysema, and tracheostomized patients with poliomyelitis, J.A.M.A. 152:1109, 1953.

Unger, L., and Unger, A. H.: The use of trypsin in bronchial asthma and other respiratory conditions, Ann. Allergy 11:494, 1953.

CHAPTER 7

# Surface-active Agents

WHILE MUCOLYTICS focus their attack on mucus *viscosity,* a second class of drugs for controlling/reducing secretions exerts an effect on the *surface tension* of pulmonary secretions. These are surface-active agents; the basic concept to be understood with this group of drugs is surface tension (Fig 7–1). Essentially, surface tension is a force occurring at liquid-gas interfaces which tends to hold the liquid surface intact. Since the liquid's molecules mutually attract (as seen in Fig 7–1), the typically rounded, or droplet, form results. Surface tension as a force is measured in dynes per centimeter, which is the force required to overcome the surface tension and cause a one-centimeter tear in the liquid surface.

The surface tension of the liquid alveolar lining is regulated by surfactant, which lowers surface tension in alveoli at low volumes and allows surface tension to increase at high lung volumes when the surfactant is "thinned." With the mucus lining of the conductive airways, *viscosity*—not surface tension—is more likely to become a problem. There is one situation, however, when surface-active agents are indicated—with frothy, bubbly pulmonary secretions. This type of secretion interferes with gas exchange, and therefore with oxygenation in the lung. In addition, the lungs are extremely difficult to clear, either by suction catheter or cough, in the frothy state. Such secretions are most likely to occur with pulmonary edema, where plasma fluid is exuded across the alveolocapillary membrane, into alveoli and small airways. In order to clear these secretions, it is imperative to reduce them to a more consistent, liquid state which can then be aspirated or expectorated.

Laplace's law states that the pressure inside a bubble is directly proportional to the surface tension of the bubble's liquid:

$$\text{pressure} = \frac{4 \times \text{surface tension}}{\text{radius}}$$

77

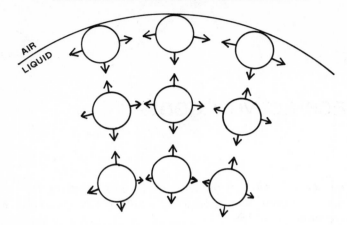

- OCCURS AT INTERFACE (LIQUID-AIR) AND IS THE FORCE EXERTED BY

MOLECULES MOVING AWAY FROM THE SURFACE, TOWARD THE CENTER OF A LIQUID.

**Fig 7–1.**—Representation of intermolecular attraction at an air-liquid interface, creating the force known as surface tension.

This can be visualized as in Figure 7–2, where a certain surface tension exists at each of the two interfaces. Since surface tension is the force holding the bubble surface intact, the pressure inside the bubble would do one of two things if surface tension were altered:

1. With *lowered* surface tension, the bubble would pop, subsiding into liquid.
2. With *increased* surface tension, the bubble would collapse, compressing the internal volume.

Generally, any agent which is used to lower surface tensions is called a *detergent.* The term "wetting agent" has sometimes been used, since soap detergents allow one to "wet down" grease by lowering its surface tension, with resulting removal facilitated. In respiratory therapy pharmacology, the term "wetting agent" can be misleading because it is easily confused with humidifying agents (mucolytics). Terminology aside, detergents in respiratory therapy are thought to *lower* the surface tension of secretions by having a lower surface tension of their own *relative* to the secretions. The term *relative* is stressed because the same end effect—liquefied, non-bubbly secretions—would result if the agents possessed high enough surface tensions relative to the secretions. Lowered surface tension is more likely.

## LAPLACE'S LAW

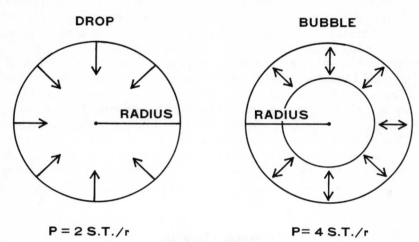

Fig 7–2.—Sketch of a bubble illustrating Laplace's law for surface tension (*S.T.*) with two liquid-air interfaces.

## SPECIFIC SURFACE-ACTIVE AGENTS

### Alcohol (ethanol, ethyl alcohol)

IDENTIFICATION: a chemical substance of relatively low surface tension.

STRENGTH: 30–50% alcohol recommended.

DOSAGE: 5–15 ml by aerosol.

MODE OF ACTION: Alcohol is thought to lower the surface tension of secretions, which results in condensation of frothy, bubbly secretions to promote expectoration and/or aspiration by suction. Frothy sputum is estimated to have a surface tension of approximately 60 dynes/cm. Alcohol has the following surface tensions at different concentrations:

> 22 dynes/cm at 100% alcohol
> 28 dynes/cm at 50% alcohol
> 32 dynes/cm at 30% alcohol

If the estimate of surface tension for frothy secretions is accurate, then alcohol would in effect lower the overall surface tension of the resulting mixture when the alcohol and the froth interact. The lowered surface tension would cause the frothy bubbles to become unstable, and the bubbles could be reduced to a liquid state. A liquid state makes aspiration then possible. The rationale for the use of vodka in an aerosol treatment is the same as that for alcohol, since vodka is a relatively pure form of alcohol.

HAZARDS: Several potential hazards may be seen with the use of alcohol by aerosol. First, mucosal irritation may occur because of direct contact of the alcohol with the respiratory mucosa. For this reason short periods of treatment are recommended when using the aerosol. A second hazard is the possibility of a slight intoxication of the patient. A third potential hazard would be due to the use of an inappropriate form of alcohol, such as isopropyl or denatured alcohol. Contraindicated in patients on Antabuse therapy for alcoholism.

## Tyloxapol (Alevaire)

IDENTIFICATION: a detergent or surface-active agent.

STRENGTH: tyloxapol (Superinone), 0.125%; bicarbonate, 2.0%; glycerin, 5.0%.

DOSAGE: 2–5 ml by aerosol.

MODE OF ACTION: Tyloxapol is thought to reduce the surface tension of secretions as alcohol does. Some investigators feel that the control of secretions resulting from the use of this compound is due to the bicarbonate reducing viscosity, more than to the action of tyloxapol. The glycerin additive is an emollient and a solvent which is added for stability of the aerosol.

HAZARDS: Hazards are rare with this drug, although bronchospasm may result, probably because of aerosol irritation in hyperreactive airways. The drug may be used with a bronchodilator additive.

NOTE: The use of glycerin as an aerosol stabilizer is preferred to that of propylene glycol. Propylene glycol is used for its hygroscopic property to prevent aerosol evaporation and shrinkage, and to promote deposition. This agent has formerly been used with a 10% saline (hyperosmolar) solution for sputum induction. Unfortunately propylene glycol was found to inhibit the growth of *Mycobacterium tuberculosis,* which is the causative agent in tuberculosis. Thus, the presence of the bacterium in the sputum culture was masked.

## Sodium ethasulfate (Tergemist)

The compound Tergemist contained 0.125% sodium ethasulfate and 0.1% potassium iodide. It has been rated ineffective, although it was intended to lower the viscosity and surface tension of secretions. The drug is no longer available for use.

## CLINICAL CONSIDERATION OF SURFACE-ACTIVE AGENTS

Surface-active agents have been used interchangeably with mucolytics in clinical practice. The technical difference between mucolytics and surface-active agents, however, lies in the basic effect: mucolytics lower *viscosity* to reduce the tenacity of secretions; surface-active agents act upon the *surface tension* of the secretions to reduce frothy or foamy secretions to a more liquid, and therefore, controllable, state. There is no evidence that surface-active agents are helpful in controlling viscous mucous secretions. The reason for this lies in the sources of foamy secretions and mucous secretions.

The classic clinical situation producing foamy secretions is acute, fulminating pulmonary edema, which can be secondary to a variety of causes, either cardiogenic or noncardiogenic. Unlike mucoid secretions which are produced by mucosal glands, the foamy secretions of pulmonary edema are thought to be derived from plasma fluid leaking across alveolocapillary membranes. This fluid can lower surfactant, causing decreased compliance and increased work of breathing, and reduce the diffusion of gases across the alveolar membrane. In addition, the foamy, bubbly nature of the fluid makes it extremely difficult for the patient or clinician to clear the airways. The resulting hypoxemia necessitates prompt treatment to improve gas exchange and prevent complications secondary to the hypoxemia.

It must be realized from the context of the pathology and the effect of surface-active agents that these agents can *only* modify the secretions themselves; i.e., the agents may lower the surface tension of the fluid to produce liquefaction. Surface-active agents do *not* treat the *cause* of the foamy fluid, which may be left ventricular failure, mitral stenosis, or irritant gas inhalation. Because of this, surface-active agents are most useful in the initial treatment to control the foamy secretions and clear the airway. More definitive therapy—such as diuretics, cardiotonics, corticosteroids (for anti-inflammation with noxious gas irritation), and fluid intake control—is utilized to deal with the *causes* and potential *sequelae* of the pulmonary edema. Chronic, routine use of surface-active agents would be unusual, since pulmonary edema is not a chronic clinical entity, and since surface-active agents would not be helpful with mucous secretions which may be of a chronic nature.

## REFERENCES

Barton, A. D.: Aerosolized detergents and mucolytic agents in the treatment of stable chronic obstructive pulmonary disease, Am. Rev. Respir. Dis. 110:104, 1974.

Clements, J. A.: Lung surfactant: Present status and future prospects, Proc. R. Soc. Med. 66:389, 1973.

Esteban, A., et al.: Continuous positive pressure ventilation in the management of eight cases of acute pulmonary oedema, Br. J. Anaesth. 45:1070, 1973.

Krishnan, B., et al.: Effect of alcohol on lung surfactant, Indian J. Exp. Biol. 11:140, 1973.

Kuz'mina, E. G., et al.: Effect of injection of synthetic detergent into the trachea and lung on basic pulmonary functions and surface tension of lung extracts, Bull. Exp. Biol. Med. 77:470, 1974.

Lyun, W. S., et al.: Composition and function of pulmonary surfactant, Ann. N.Y. Acad. Sci. 221:209, 1974.

Miller, J. B., et al.: Alevaire inhalation for eliminating secretions in asthmatic sinusitis, bronchiectasis and bronchitis of adults, Ann. Allergy, 12:611, 1954.

Modell, J. H., et al.: The effects of wetting and antifoaming agents on pulmonary surfactant, Anesthesiology, 30:164, 1969.

Paez, P. N., and Miller, W. F.: Surface active agents in sputum evacuation: A blind comparison with normal saline solution and distilled water, Chest 60:312, 1971.

Palmer, K. N. V.: Effect of an aerosol detergent in chronic bronchitis, Lancet, 1:611, 1957.

Petrov, O. V.: A method of measuring the surface tension and surface potential of lung surfactants, Bull. Exp. Biol. Med. 77:210, 1974.

Reifenrath, R., et al.: Surface tension properties of lung alveolar surfactant obtained by alveolar micropuncture, Respir. Physiol. 19:369, 1973.

Tainter, M. L., et al.: Alevaire as a mucolytic agent, N. Engl. J. Med. 253:764, 1955.

# CHAPTER 8

# Corticosteroids in Respiratory Therapy

CORTICOSTEROIDS represent one of the most physiologically interesting and complex group of drugs in pharmacology. By way of a comprehensive preview, it can be said that glucocorticoids, or "steroids" as they are commonly called, have three major pharmacologic effects:

1. Bronchodilation, either direct, or indirect through potentiation, of beta sympathomimetics;
2. Anti-inflammation;
3. Immunosuppression.

Because of these first two effects, corticosteroids have been of value in treating or controlling asthma, especially the intrinsic, nonallergic type where hyposensitization is not an alternative. They have also played a role in treating allergic, extrinsic asthma when other measures prove inadequate. Therapy with corticosteroids, however, is fraught with potential hazards and therefore requires complete and careful understanding by clinicians. To understand these and other effects of corticosteroids, it is necessary to review their role and source in the body.

Generally, body function of any sort is controlled by two major systems: the nervous system and the endocrine (hormonal) system. The nervous system is composed of the central and peripheral branches of neuron branchings (see Chapter 3). The second, the endocrine, is composed of the various glands and organs which secrete hormones, such as the thyroid gland, the pancreas, the testes or ovaries. The two control systems often form an interrelated complex, with neural impulses triggering the release of hormones by glands. For example, the hypothalamus under certain conditions will stimulate an area above the pituitary gland (see Fig 8–6) known as the median eminence, which will, in turn, secrete a chemical termed corticotropin-releasing factor. Thus nervous inpulses can trigger the release of hormones.

*Hormone:* a chemical substance secreted into the body fluids by one or more cells to exert a physiologic effect on other cells of the body.

Usually hormones are distributed by the vascular system, an important factor in the time of onset and duration of effect. In general, hormonal, or endocrine, control performs slower, more regulatory functions of metabolism contrasted with the speed of nervous control.

## ANATOMY AND PHYSIOLOGY OF CORTICOSTEROIDS

Corticosteroids are hormones secreted by the adrenal cortex. The adrenal glands are small organs located on top of each kidney, as shown in Figure 8–1. A cross section of the adrenal gland reveals an inner area known as the medulla, with many chromaffin granules, and an outer zone known as the cortex.

In reality, the adrenal glands, or suprarenal glands as they are also termed, are a combination of two functionally distinct glands:

*Adrenal medulla:* the inner zone, or smaller portion of the adrenal gland; pale pink in a fresh specimen. There is no connective tissue barrier between the cortex and the medulla, but an actual intermingling of the two types of cells for a short distance. The adrenal medulla is under sympathetic autonomic control, and can be stimulated to release epinephrine (secreted in the chromaffin granules) and some norepinephrine.

*Adrenal cortex:* the outer part of the adrenal gland. Its outermost portion is deep yellow and the inner area a dark red or brown.

**Fig 8–1.**—Location and cross section of the adrenal, or suprarenal gland.

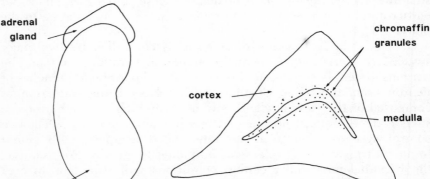

Unlike the adrenal medulla, the adrenal cortex *is* essential to life.

The adrenal cortex secretes the hormones that are necessary for body homeostasis:

*Glucocorticoids:* hormones, such as cortisol, needed to regulate metabolic rates and functions.

*Mineralocorticoids:* hormones, such as aldosterone, or corticosterone, needed to regulate body water and electrolyte concentrations ($Na^+$, $K^+$, $Cl^-$). For example, aldosterone helps to control the reabsorption of $Na^+$ and excretion of $K^+$ in renal tubules.

A comprehensive, summary overview of the adrenal gland can be given:

Adrenal gland

1. Adrenal medulla
   a. Epinephrine
   b. Norepinephrine $\Big\}$ Sympathetic nervous control
2. Adrenal cortex
   a. Corticosteroids
      (1) Mineralocorticoids, e.g., aldosterone
      (2) Glucocorticoids, e.g., cortisol
   b. Androgens

The term *steroid* is rather loosely used, since there are several major types of hormones secreted by the adrenal cortex. A more precise term is *corticosteroid* to indicate the chemical family of substances produced by the cortex, with the very specific term *glucocorticoid* reserved for the class of cortisol-like hormones. In respiratory therapy, there are three drugs falling within the glucocorticoid class:

dexamethasone sodium phosphate (Decadron)

beclomethasone dipropionate (Vanceril)

triamcinolone acetonide (not yet available)

## STRUCTURE-ACTIVITY RELATIONS OF CORTICOSTEROIDS

Such glucocorticoids are defined structurally by the common steroid nucleus, seen in the carbon skeleton (Fig 8–2).

Functionally, the variation or specificity of action among different compounds depends on the attachment of various radicals (hydrogen, hydroxyl, oxygen) at sites on the parent nucleus. For example, it is interesting that the basic anti-inflammatory action of glucocorticoids is dependent on certain essential groups attached to the nucleus at the circled locations seen in Figure 8–3.

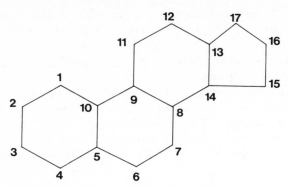

**Fig 8–2.**—Characteristic 4-ring corticosteroid nucleus.

Dexamethasone possesses enhanced anti-inflammatory properties, which makes it useful for treating chronic allergic asthmatics. Basically, dexamethasone is cortisol with an added 1,2 double bond, and other substituents (Fig 8–4). Beclomethasone has even more attachments, but the basic steroid nucleus is still quite visible, as seen in Figure 8–5.

The perspective of drug development among the glucocorticoids for use with chronic asthmatic patients is analogous to that of the beta-two sympathomimetics: in both cases, more specific agents with fewer harmful side effects are sought through continued chemical synthesis of compounds.

**Fig 8–3.**—Attachments at the *3-, 4-, 11-,* and *17-*carbon positions which are essential for the anti-inflammatory action of the glucocorticoid.

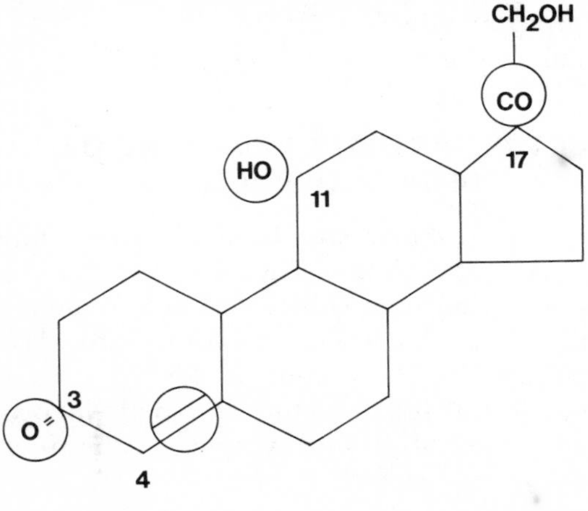

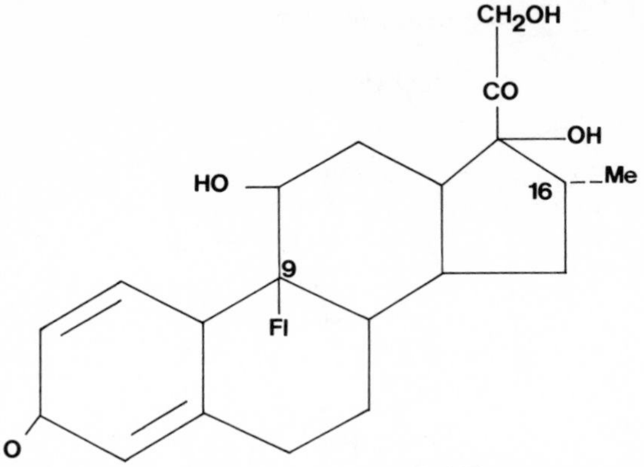

**Fig 8–4.**—Dexamethasone (16α-methyl-9α-fluoroprednisolone).

## NEUROSECRETORY CONTROL OF ADRENAL CORTEX

Essentially, glucocorticoids are released under the influence of adrenocorticotropic hormone (ACTH, or corticotropin). The full path for release and control of corticosteroids is seen in Figure 8–6.

Stimulation of the hypothalamus causes impulses to be sent to the area known as the median eminence, where corticotropin-releasing factor (CRF) is released and circulates through the portal vessel to the anterior pituitary gland. Under the influence of CRF, the anterior

**Fig 8–5.**—Beclomethasone dipropionate, the active ingredient in Vanceril Inhaler, is an anti-inflammatory corticosteroid.

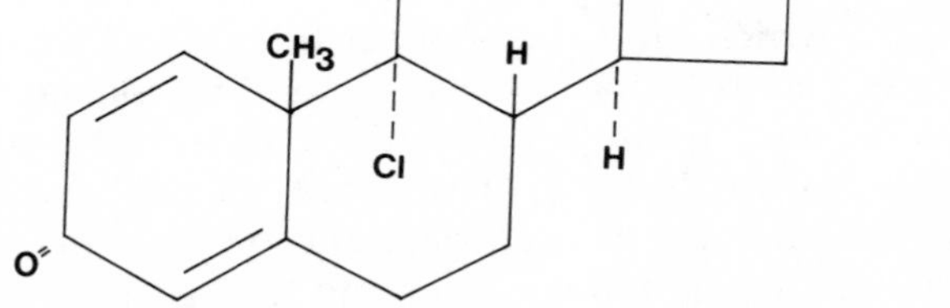

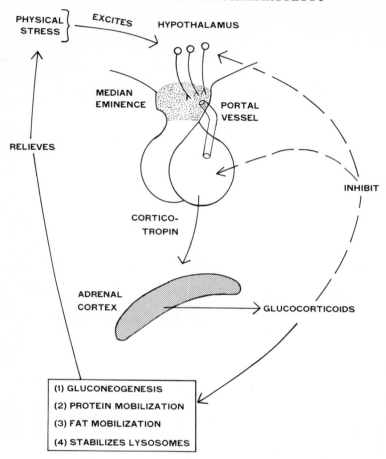

**MECHANISM FOR REGULATION OF GLUCOCORTICOID SECRETION**

**Fig 8–6.**—Physiology of corticosteroid secretion and control.

pituitary releases adrenocorticotropic hormone, or ACTH, into the bloodstream. ACTH, in turn, stimulates the adrenal cortex to secrete glucocorticoids, which alter metabolism to break down proteins for use of the amino acids in the Krebs cycle (gluconeogenesis). Metabolism of proteins and lipids is a defensive measure to increase body reserves of energy in the face of stress. A natural rhythm of stress occurs as individuals begin each day, and glucocorticoid levels are highest in the morning hours, assuming a normal nocturnal sleep cycle. The path between the hypothalamus and pituitary which controls the adrenal cortex is frequently termed the *hypothalamic-pituitary-adrenal axis* (HPA) in drug literature.

Examples of stress include trauma of any sort, heat, cold, sympathomimetics, surgery, and debilitating disease. The self-regulating feedback mechanism causes high levels of corticosteroids to depress or inhibit both the hypothalamus and the anterior pituitary. This action is of extreme importance in therapeutic use of corticosteroids.

## PHARMACOLOGY AND EFFECTS OF GLUCOCORTICOIDS

### Anti-inflammatory Effects

The major use of corticosteroids in respiratory patients is to reduce or inhibit the inflammatory type of reaction associated with asthmatics. Essentially, the inflammatory response in the lung is characterized by the pathologic triad:

1. Bronchoconstriction;
2. Increased secretions;
3. Mucosal edema.

This triple response causes the clinical symptoms of wheezing, cough, dyspnea, and measurable changes in airway resistance. The causes of irritation or trauma resulting in inflammation of lung tissue include:

1. Inhaled pollutants (dust, aerosol, noxious gases);
2. Physical/mechanical insult (catheters, foreign objects);
3. High-velocity flow rates in hyperreactive airways;
4. Mast cell degranulation releasing histamine (antigen-antibody reaction, type 1).

The schema illustrated in Figure 8–7 outlines the sequence of events resulting in inflammatory injuries.

**Fig 8–7.**—Cellular insult often results in *lysosome rupture* and *kallikrein* release, which converts certain proteins in the blood to *bradykinin,* a potent vasodilator. Corticosteroids may stabilize the lysosomal membrane to inhibit such kallikrein release and subsequent inflammation.

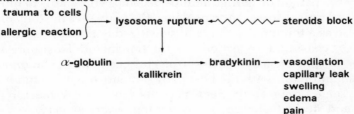

*Lysosome rupture* causes release of kallikrein, an enzyme, which converts the plasma alpha-globulin to a nonapeptide, bradykinin. This is a potent vasodilator, and causes capillary leakage of plasma-like fluid out of the capillary into the damaged area, with subsequent infiltration by leukocytes, and, ultimately, tissue healing by fibrous ingrowth. *Histamine release,* in allergy or injury, is also responsible for the inflammatory response. Although intended as a saving, defensive measure, inflammation itself can be harmful, especially when occurring in the lung. Glucocorticoids are thought to stabilize the lysosomal membrane, thus preventing or reducing the inflammatory sequence. They also affect histamine by:

1. Depleting tissue histamine;
2. Delaying histamine resynthesis;
3. Inhibiting histidine decarboxylase, the enzyme responsible for converting histidine to histamine.

## Enhanced Bronchodilation

Bronchodilation is increased either *indirectly,* by restoring responsiveness to sympathomimetics (isoproterenol), or through *direct* relaxation of bronchial smooth muscle.

## Immunosuppression

Immunosuppression is a Janus effect. One aspect is good, if immunosuppression is the desired goal, as in transplants; but another is bad, since increased risk of infection then threatens the patient. This effect is seen with large doses of glucocorticoids over prolonged periods.

At the risk of oversimplification, one can say that the body protects itself against all foreign invaders by means of the immune system. The major weapons of this system are *cellular immunity* through sensitized lymphocytes, and *humoral* (circulating) immunity through dissolved antibodies in the bloodstream. Corticosteroids can suppress the lymphocyte system which is crucial to these basic immune processes. Thereby the patient on corticosteroids becomes vulnerable to infecting agents, and thus disease. In transplants, the body sees the transplanted organ also as a foreign invader, and sensitized lymphocytes will attack the organ, causing a "rejection" of the transplant. To suppress this, patients are put on massive doses of corticosteroids. The organ can then heal and mesh with the host body, but any other foreign invader has the same opportunity. Such patients require extreme care, with asepsis and sterile technique in suctioning or airway care.

## General Physiologic Effects

Since glucocorticoids are essentially anti-insulin regulators of metabolism by causing increased hepatic synthesis of glucose (gluconeogenesis), the following effects can be seen:

1. Increased glucose, which can lead to "steroid diabetes," or loss of the insulin-regulated glucose metabolism.
2. Decreased peripheral muscle due to breakdown of protein for use in gluconeogenesis.
3. Water retention and peripheral edema due to the sodium-sparing effects of corticosteroids.
4. Increased gastric acidity with resulting stress ulcer.
5. Increased blood pressure.
6. Decreased bone calcium predisposing to fractures of the long bones.
7. Hypercorticism, or excess levels of corticosteroids, known as cushingoid effect. Patients present a general picture of moon face, humpback, thin arms and legs, and pedal edema.
8. Adrenal suppression—due to high levels of exogenous steroids.

## Diurnal Rhythms and Alternate-Day Therapy

Normally, ACTH and cortisol levels in the body rise and fall on a daily basis in coordination with the schedule needs of the body rather than remaining constant. This daily rhythm is termed *diurnal* or *circadian,* and is visualized in Figure 8–8.

Cortisol peaks about the time one awakens, to aid in meeting the stressful needs of beginning the day's activities, with its metabolic functions. Likewise, cortisol reaches a low at approximately midnight, when it again starts building. The level of cortisol is secondary to the level of ACTH, which peaks and falls just ahead of the cortisol (see

**Fig 8–8.**—Diurnal variations in ACTH (dotted curve), and cortisol (solid curve).

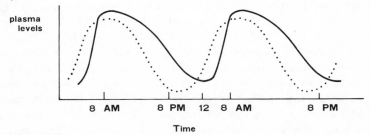

"Neurosecretory Control of Adrenal Cortex," this chapter). The rhythm pictured assumes a normal daytime work schedule, with nighttime sleeping. Reversed schedules for night workers simply allow the same rhythm on a different schedule. It does require time for the body to adjust to new schedules, however—a factor noted in jet lag and the initial difficulty in adjusting to a night shift.

Because a feedback mechanism exists by which high levels of ACTH and cortisol inhibit further release of these same agents, pharmacologic administration of steroids can upset the usual diurnal rhythm. For example, giving doses of a corticosteroid in the afternoon or evening deceives the body into suppression of its own ACTH-cortisol secretion and exposes tissues to abnormal levels of steroids. Adrenal suppression and hypercorticism with loss of endogenous corticosteroids can result, as well as tissue side effects of edema, and cushingoid symptoms.

Alternate-day therapy mimics the natural diurnal rhythm by giving a steroid drug early in the morning, when normal tissue levels are high. Thus, suppression of the hypothalamic-pituitary-adrenal system occurs at the same time it normally would occur with the body's own steroid, and, on the alternate day, the regular diurnal secretion in the hypothalamic-pituitary-adrenal (HPA) system can resume. Tissue side effects are minimized since the drug is administered at the time when tissues are normally exposed to high corticosteroid levels by the body's rhythm. Use of an intermediate-acting corticosteroid drug, with duration of 12–36 hours, allows drug therapy to be restricted to alternate days so that peak exposure of tissues is further minimized.

## Aerosol vs Oral Therapy

Attempts to use aerosolized corticosteroids with chronic asthmatics who required steroid therapy were reported as early as 1951. The aerosol route of administration represented an effort to treat the airways without the systemic side effects of adrenal suppression or cushingoid symptoms (moon face, edema, humpback). Cortisone, hydrocortisone, prednisone, and finally dexamethasone were all tried between 1951 and 1963, but although all produced the anticipated therapeutic effect of improved airway resistance, each unfortunately caused hypercorticism and adrenal suppression. Until 1976, dexamethasone remained the aerosolizable steroid of choice despite this fact. In each agent, the therapeutic dose was large enough to lead to systemic absorption, with the resulting side effects. Because of this, aerosolized steroids have not proven particularly useful over the oral route for long-term administration, where systemic side effects are so difficult to control or prevent. But it is precisely because of this situation that several new steroids have renewed the exciting possibilities for aerosol administration. These are beclomethasone dipropionate (Vanceril), which was recently approved for use in the United States, and triamcinolone acetonide (not yet available). The promise of both drugs lies in the fact that the therapeutic dose by aerosol causes minimal systemic absorption, and this prevents the undesired side effects while controlling hyperreactive airways.

## SPECIFIC AEROSOL CORTICOSTEROIDS

### Dexamethasone sodium phosphate (Decadron)

IDENTIFICATION: long-acting, anti-inflammatory, synthetic analogue of cortisol.

STRENGTH: 12.6 gram cartridge, per metered spray: 0.1 mg dexamethasone phosphate plus fluorochlorohydrocarbons as propellants and 2% alcohol.

DOSAGE: usually determined by physician.

MODE OF ACTION: basic anti-inflammatory effect thought to be due to lysosomal stabilization, which prevents the release of kallikrein, an enzyme converting alpha-globulins (protein kininogens, or precursors of bradykinin) to bradykinin. Bradykinin, in turn, causes capillary leaking, pain, and edema. Lysosome rupture may be due to trauma or irritants, including that released by mast cell discharge of histamine with *its* subsequent trauma. There is some evidence that corticosteroids either enhance beta responsiveness or directly relax smooth muscle in the airway, or both. Restored beta response would also retard mast cell release of mediators, because of increased cyclic AMP in response to endogenous epinephrine levels.

HAZARDS: The plasma half-life of dexamethasone is approximately 200 minutes. However, the tissue effects, termed biologic half-life, initiated by the drug, persist up to 72 hours. Such long-acting drugs are more likely to produce cushingoid side effects because of the persistent round-the-clock stimulation of tissues. Therefore, hazards include all of the side effects of steroids: adrenal suppression, water retention, muscle wasting, hypertension, and risk of impaired immune response. Unfortunately, all of these effects are possible since the therapeutic dose of dexamethasone leads to some system absorption even when given by aerosol.

   If adrenal suppression *has* occurred, termination of dexamethasone represents a hazard, since the lack of natural steroids will be detrimental before adrenal secretion resumes.

## Beclomethasone dipropionate (Vanceril)

IDENTIFICATION: a long-acting, anti-inflammatory steroid; synthetic, chemically related to prednisolone, with a chlorine at the 9-alpha and a methyl group at the 16-beta position (see "Structure-Activity Relations of Corticosteroids," this chapter).

STRENGTH: 10 mg inhaler canister. Each actuation gives approximately 50 μg of beclomethasone. There are 200 oral inhalations per inhaler.

DOSAGE: The usual dose is 2 inhalations (100 μg), 3–4 times per day. A starting dose of 12–16 inhalations per day, subsequently adjusted downward, is suggested. Maximum intake per day should not exceed 1,000 μg (20 inhalations).

MODE OF ACTION: The basic effect of this drug is anti-inflammatory, which may be mediated through the cyclic AMP pathway, causing inhibited mast cell release as well as lysosome stabilization. There is a possibility of enhanced beta responsiveness to endogenous epinephrine in the body and/or direct relaxation of the bronchial smooth muscle. Pre-clinical tests showed that the conventional dose of 400 μg per day exerted as much benefit as up to 1,600 μg. There were no systemic side effects or adrenal suppression noted with this dosage. A maximum dose of 2 mg/day produced therapeutic effects also, but has been noted to produce adrenal suppression.

HAZARDS: Patients formerly on systemic steroids for control of bronchial asthma may die of adrenal insufficiency when transferred to aerosol beclomethasone, since this drug does not provide systemic levels of the steroid. A number of months may be required before hypothalamic-pituitary-adrenal axis function is recovered, with supplementary steroids needed during this time. Beclomethasone is contraindicated as a primary treatment of status asthmaticus. This drug is not a bronchodilator. It should not be used for the acute relief of bronchospasm. The potential effects of beclomethasone on pulmonary infections are not known. Systemic infection due to immunosuppression is not a problem since there is no evidence of systemic absorption with the therapeutic dose required by the aerosol route of administration.

## Triamcinolone acetonide

Triamcinolone acetonide has not been released for general clinical use in the United States, and the American manufacturer has been experiencing some instability problems with the agent. Triamcinolone is a non-polar, water-insoluble compound, prepared in a Freon-powered aerosol cartridge, with an adapter for small airway deposition designed to deliver 90% of the particles less than 5 microns in diameter. Trial doses of 0.9 mg per day resulted in an increased maximal expiratory flow rate. Plasma cortisol levels during maximal dosage of the drug (2 mg per day) remained normal, thereby indicating poor systemic absorption.

Both triamcinolone and beclomethasone are of great use by the aerosol route of administration since both can produce therapeutic effects in asthmatic patients (increased flow rates, decreased airway resistance, anti-inflammatory action) without evidence of the systemic absorption which has previously been a problem with the aerosol administration of steroids, such as dexamethasone.

## REFERENCES

Aviado, D. M., and Carrillo, L. R.: Anti-asthmatic action of corticosteroids: A review of the literature on their mechanism of action, J. Clin. Pharmacol. 10:3, 1970.

Cronin, M. P.: Steroids in respiratory therapy, Respir. Ther. 5:33, 1975.

Fauci, A. S., et al.: Glucocorticosteroid therapy: Mechanisms of action and clinical considerations, Ann. Intern. Med. 84:304, 1976.

Godfrey, S.: The place of a new aerosol steroid, beclomethasone dipropionate, in the management of childhood asthma, Pediatr. Clin. North Am. 22:147, 1975.

Symposium on steroid therapy, Med. Clin. North Am., 57, (Sept.) 1973, especially the following articles: Bacon, G. E. and Spencer, M. L.: Pediatric uses of steroids, pp. 1265–76. Dale, D. C., and Petersdorf, R. G.: Corticosteroids and infectious diseases, pp. 1277–87. Dluhy, R. G., Lauler, D. P., and Thorn, G. W.: Pharmacology and chemistry of adrenal glucocorticoids, pp. 1155–65. Kirkpatrick, C. H.: Steroid therapy of allergic diseases, pp. 1309–20. Zurier, R. B., and Weissmann, G.: Anti-immunologic and anti-inflammatory effects of steroid therapy, pp. 1295–1307.

CHAPTER **9**

# Cromolyn Sodium: Antiasthmatic

IN JANUARY OF 1965, a bischromone, later known as cromolyn sodium, was synthesized in the Fisons laboratory, and demonstrated the ability to prevent bronchospasm in an asthmatic volunteer. This drug, a synthetic derivative of khellin, the active ingredient found in the Mediterranean plant *Ammi visnaga,* was first introduced in Britain in 1968, and is now available for use in the United States.

In order to understand the mode of action with cromolyn sodium, a brief review of asthma, and allergic reaction, is required.

## PHYSIOLOGY OF ALLERGIC ASTHMA

Bronchial asthma is a usually reversible, intermittent, narrowing of the airways, with increased secretions and possibly edema of the mucous lining. When the pathology exists, wheezing, cough, dyspnea, and often hypoxemia are confirming symptoms.

Asthma has been distinguished into two types on the basis of etiology:

1. Extrinsic, allergic, atopic—This type of asthma is a true sensitivity, or allergy, to certain substances, involving antigen-antibody reaction with subsequent pulmonary inflammatory response. Antigens include pollen, foods, dander, etc.
2. Intrinsic, nonallergic, non-atopic—In addition to antigen-mediated asthma, another type of asthma exists which has no clear-cut, single cause. Predisposing situations include anxiety, aerosols, dust, infection, or exercise.

Beta blockade, or a general unresponsiveness to endogenous epinephrine and norepinephrine levels, has been used to explain intrinsic, nonallergic bronchoconstriction, and even extended as a causative factor in the histamine release of allergic asthma, although antigenic stimulation remains the primary etiologic factor. Schematically, in early studies this was seen as a common, physiologic pathway of bronchoconstriction (Fig 9–1).

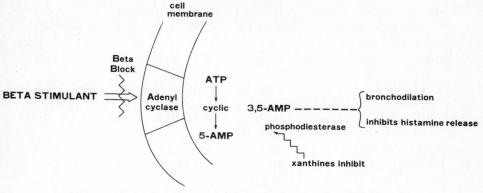

**Fig 9–1.**—Beta pathway and physiologic effects of cyclic AMP.

More recent research indicates that bronchospasm and constriction are a result of nucleotide imbalance (cyclic AMP–cyclic GMP balance), whether caused by antigen stimulation, beta unresponsiveness, irritation of vagal receptors, or overactive alpha stimulation. This view was explored in Chapter 3.

In terms of respiratory pharmacology, there is a specific agent—cromolyn sodium—used to control allergic, extrinsic asthma; corticosteroids have been reviewed previously as useful for anti-inflammatory effects with both types of asthma (intrinsic and extrinsic). Since cromolyn sodium is especially directed at extrinsic, allergic asthma, a brief consideration of the allergic response in the lung is needed.

The term *atopy* means a sensitivity to foreign, antigenic substances, in the form of antibody buildup following antigen exposure. The allergic response in asthma is essentially an immune response—and a *mistaken* response at that, somewhat akin to a military guard firing at a stray cow in a war zone instead of at the real enemy.

There are basically two branches of the immune response: sensitized lymphocytes (cellular immunity); and circulating antibodies (humoral immunity).

*Cellular immunity* is responsible for tissue rejection in transplants as well as the PPD (purified protein derivative) reaction in the skin test for tuberculosis exposure. This is termed a type 4, or delayed, type of hypersensitivity.

*Humoral immunity* is involved in allergic asthma, as well as the routine protection of the body against mumps, measles, polio, and other disease.

*Antigen:* a substance which is capable of provoking antibodies and/or cellular immunity when administered to an immunologically competent animal.

*Antibody:* a serum globulin or protein, modified to combine and react with its specific antigen.

Antibodies are also called immunoglobulins. There are approximately 30 serum proteins, such as albumin, and of these, 5 are immunoglobulins, or substances capable of becoming specific antibodies. Immunoglobulins are grouped as follows:

immunoglobulin G, IgG, 80% ⎫
immunoglobulin A, IgA, 10% ⎬  major class
immunoglobulin M, IgM, 5–10% ⎭
immunoglobulin D, IgD, trace ⎫  minor class
immunoglobulin E, IgE, trace ⎭

IgG is the antibody most responsible for protection against the common diseases usually encountered in growing up, which is why the clinical condition of agammaglobulinemia (lack of gammaglobulin, IgG) is life-threatening.

IgA exists as serum IgA and secretory IgA, probably playing an important role in protecting the respiratory tract from infecting viruses or bacteria. IgA is found in salivary as well as bronchial secretions, tears, human milk, and the GI tract. Secretory IgA is characterized by the presence of a *secretory piece* which is thought to provide resistance to degradation by proteolytic enzymes (Fig 9–2).

Secretory IgA guards against respiratory tract infections such as influenza, poliovirus, or rhinovirus. Patients who lack respiratory tract IgA experience recurrent pulmonary infections. Since the lung is essentially open to a contaminated environment, IgA provides a first line of defense.

Antibodies offer defense against invading organisms by being specific to the organism. The basic sequence is exposure to an organism

**Fig 9–2.**—Secretory IgA.

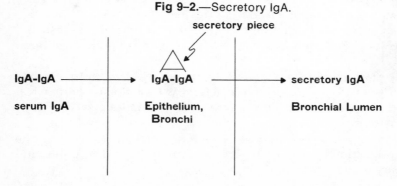

(virus, etc.), with specific antibody developing against that organism, and then, upon re-exposure, the antibody will react specifically with the organism (Fig 9–3). This antigen-antibody reaction *inactivates* or kills the organism, preventing any disease resulting from the exposure to the organism.

IgE has been the antibody of interest for allergic asthma ever since this substance was discovered and studied by Ishizaka in 1966. IgE is also known as reagin, or reaginic antibody. The role of IgE is basic to the allergic response, as outlined here:

first exposure to antigen, e.g., pollen, ragweed
↓
production of IgE specific to the antigen
↓
re-exposure to antigen
↓
antigen-antibody reaction
↓
symptoms of inflammation

(wheeze, runny nose, cough, etc.)

**Fig 9–3.**—Antibody formation with subsequent antigen-antibody reaction.

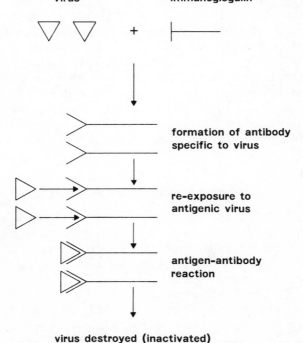

virus destroyed (inactivated)

In slightly more detail, IgE is a circulating, or humoral, immunoglobulin, but once it is *sensitized,* or made specific to a certain antigen, it will attach to cells known as *mast cells.* The term *cytophilic antibody* describes this affinity of IgE for cell surfaces. Mast cells are specialized cells found in the lung, located primarily in clusters around peribronchial nerve and vascular areas. The mast cell is a storehouse of mediators of inflammation, such as histamine, heparin (possibly), slow-reacting substance of anaphylaxis (SRS-A) and eosinophilic chemotactic factor of anaphylaxis (ECF-A), and serotonin (not found in human mast cells). As such, the cell is analogous to a loaded gun, since these mediators cause the inflammatory response of bronchoconstriction and obstructing secretions in asthma. Everyone has mast cells, in both lungs and skin tissue; *allergic individuals* however, build up IgE levels which attach to the mast cell. The analogous gun is now cocked. Re-exposure to the antigen, i.e., to the substance to which one is allergic, causes the antigen to interact with the IgE on the cell surface. Bridging of the IgE by the antigen, in turn, stimulates the mast cell to discharge granules of the inflammatory mediators. This is represented in Figure 9–4.

There is interesting evidence that mast cell discharge, or degranulation as it is also known, is controlled by the autonomic nervous system through the cyclic AMP–cyclic GMP nucleotides. Briefly, increased AMP levels can retard mast cell degranulation and inflammation, and GMP enhances this effect. This is why beta blockade *can* increase histamine release of extrinsic, allergic asthmatics, although the immediate cause is the antigen exposure. Of course beta blockade *without* antigen, and IgE-mediated release of inflammatory substances, can also cause bronchoconstriction because of the drop in AMP levels. The entire scheme of nervous regulation through the nucleotides in relation to histamine release (i.e., mast cell discharge) can be seen in Figure 9–5.

### Cromolyn sodium (Intal, Aarane)

IDENTIFICATION: The bischromone, cromolyn sodium, is a synthetic derivative of khellin, an active ingredient extracted from the Mediterranean plant *Ammi visnaga.* The synthetic derivative eliminates the side effects of nausea and vomiting found with khellin.

STRENGTH: 20 mg capsules.

DOSAGE: 1 capsule in Spin-haler 4 times daily (Spin-haler is a device for puncturing the capsule and inhaling the powder contained within). There is no pressurized cartridge or Freon-type of propel-

## TARGET CELL ACTIVATION,
## MEDIATOR GENERATION AND RELEASE

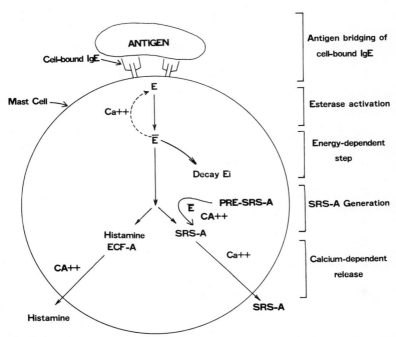

**Fig 9–4.**—Sequence of events leading to mediator release from the mast cell in allergic asthma. (Adapted from Austen, K. F., and Orange, R. P.: Am. Rev. Respir. Dis. 112:423, 1975.)

lant with the Spin-haler. The patient inhales the powder contained in the capsule, after the capsule is punctured. This route of administration was chosen because of the limited solubility of the drug, and the large 20 mg dose required, which precluded the use of a conventional aerosol.

MODE OF ACTION: Cromolyn sodium is thought to inhibit the degranulation of mast cells during the antigen-antibody reactions, thereby preventing the release of the chemical mediators of inflammation such as histamine, heparin, SRS-A. The drug does not affect autonomic pathways nor act through the cyclic AMP–cyclic GMP system. IgE levels in asthmatic patients remain high, indicating that antibody formation is not blocked. The overall mode of action is seen in Figure 9–6. Because of the mode of action, cromolyn sodium must be viewed as a prophylactic agent in the treatment of

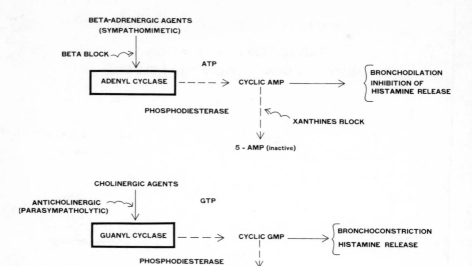

**Fig 9–5.**—Pathways of cyclic AMP–cyclic GMP control and release. A more detailed treatment is given in Chapter 3.

**Fig 9–6.**—Basic mechanism and site of action of cromolyn sodium.

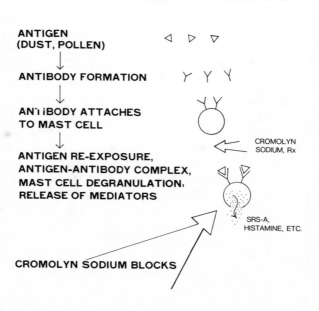

asthma. There is no solid evidence that it exerts a direct broncho-dilating effect, or that it otherwise acts on bronchial smooth muscle. Consequently, it should not be used as a treatment of choice during episodes of acute bronchospasm.

HAZARDS: Bronchospasm is a hazard with aerosol inhalation of the drug powder, probably because of local epithelial irritation, with resulting parasympathetic (vagus-induced) constriction.

## REFERENCES

Anand, S. C., and Goodman, D. H.: Protective effect of cromolyn sodium on bronchial challenge tests in pollen asthma, Ann. Allergy 30:64, 1972.

Assem, E. S. K., and Mongar, J. L.: Inhibition of allergic reactions in man and other species by cromoglycate, Int. Arch. Allergy Appl. Immunol. 38:68, 1970.

Austen, K. F., and Lichtenstein, L. M. (eds.): *Asthma: Physiology, Immuno-pharmacology and Treatment* (New York: Academic Press, 1973).

Austen, K. F., and Orange, R. P.: Bronchial asthma: The possible role of the chemical mediators of immediate hypersensitivity in the pathogenesis of subacute chronic disease, Am. Rev. Respir. Dis. 112:423, 1975.

Falliers, C. J.: Cromolyn sodium (disodium cromoglycate) prophylaxis, Pediatr. Clin. North Am. 22:141, 1975.

Gross, G. N., Souhadra, J. F., and Farr, R. S.: The long-term treatment of an asthmatic patient using phentolamine, Chest 66:397, 1974.

*Intal (Cromolyn sodium—Fisons)* (Bedford, Mass.: Fisons Corp., 1973).

Nelson, H. S.: The beta adrenergic theory of bronchial asthma, Pediatr. Clin. North Am. 22:53, 1975.

Orr, T. S. C.: Mast cells and allergic asthma, Br. J. Dis. Chest 67:87, 1973.

Parker, W. A.: Cromolyn sodium, Respir. Care 19:529, 1974.

Reed, C. E.: The pathogenesis of asthma, Med. Clin. North Am. 58:55, 1974.

Said, S. I.: The lung in relation to vasoactive hormones, Fed. Proc. 32:1972, 1973.

The Immune System, Am. J. Nurs. 76:1614, 1976 (a special section of several articles devoted to immune response and clinical application).

# CHAPTER 10

# Antibiotics in Respiratory Therapy

ANTIBIOTICS have proved to be one of the most useful, and most used, class of drugs in modern therapeutics.

*Antibiotic:* a substance, produced by microorganisms (bacteria, fungi, molds), which is capable of inhibiting or killing bacteria and other microorganisms.

## HISTORY

The classic discovery of penicillin by Fleming in 1928 led to further research for the isolation and identification of additional antibiotics. The definition above was offered by Waksman in 1941. Since then, antibiotics have been produced synthetically in the laboratory, as is the case with most drugs, and thus requiring some expansion of the original definition to include laboratory origin of antibiotic substances.

## MODES OF ACTION

The following mechanisms by which antibiotics inhibit or kill microorganisms have been identified or postulated:

1. INHIBITION OF CELL WALL SYNTHESIS: Bacteria possess rigid cell walls, unlike many other cells which have only a membrane. This wall is needed to protect the bacterial cell because of high internal osmotic pressures. Without this protection, in the *relatively* hypotonic environment of the body, such cells will explode. Examples of antibiotics are penicillins, bacitracin, cephalosporins, vancomycin, and cycloserine.
2. INHIBITION OF CELL MEMBRANE FUNCTION: The cytoplasmic membrane which encloses a cell is a very selective, functional, active filter to keep certain proteins and nucleotides within the cell and to allow other substances to enter the cell for metabolism.

Disruption of the membrane function upsets the necessary flow and storage of cell material required for growth or life. The membrane of certain bacteria and fungi are especially susceptible to particular antibiotics, such as, for example, the polymyxins.

3. INHIBITION OF PROTEIN SYNTHESIS: Protein synthesis is crucial to a cell's growth and function, because amino acids are linked to produce protein for structural enlargement, energy storage, or enzymes. Many antibiotics interfere with the ribosome's ability to synthesize needed proteins. Examples are chloramphenicol, tetracyclines, erythromycin, lincomycin, streptomycin, kanamycin, and gentamicin; the last three are aminoglycosides.

4. INHIBITION OF NUCLEIC ACID SYNTHESIS: DNA synthesis is the center of cellular activity and life, acting as the master code for cell function and structure. Certain antibiotics will attach to the DNA strands and block further DNA replication or formation of messenger RNA. Examples are actinomycin, mitomycins, and rifampin.

## CLINICAL ASPECTS OF ANTIBIOTICS

In general, antibiotics can be either *bactericidal* or *bacteriostatic,* depending on the particular drug and mode of action. Examples of both types of antibiotics are listed in Table 10–1.

Antibiotics are also distinguished as broad spectrum or narrow spectrum:

Broad-spectrum antibiotic: useful against a wide range of organisms, both gram-positive and gram-negative bacteria.

Narrow-spectrum antibiotic: useful against only a few organisms. See Table 10–2 for examples of each spectrum of activity.

Antibiotics are tested for use in therapy through sensitivity and

TABLE 10–1.  EXAMPLES OF BACTERICIDAL AND BACTERIOSTATIC ANTIBIOTICS.

| BACTERICIDAL ANTIBIOTICS | BACTERIOSTATIC ANTIBIOTICS |
| --- | --- |
| Penicillins | Chloramphenicol |
| Cephalosporins | Erythromycin |
| Cycloserine | Tetracyclines |
| Vancomycin | Lincomycin |
| Bacitracin | |
| Streptomycin | |
| Kanamycin | |
| Polymyxins | |

TABLE 10–2.   EXAMPLES OF BROAD-SPECTRUM AND
NARROW-SPECTRUM ANTIBIOTICS

| BROAD | NARROW |
|---|---|
| Chloramphenicol | Penicillin |
| Tetracyclines | Streptomycin |
| Kanamycin | Erythromycin |
| Cephalosporins | Lincomycin |
| Ampicillin | Polymyxin B |
| | Vancomycin |

resistance (S & R) studies. Various antibiotics are impregnated onto disks of filter paper, and placed in dishes, with each dish heavily inoculated with a different bacterial agent (Fig 10–1). If the organism is susceptible, or sensitive, to the antibiotic on a particular disk, then a clear zone of inhibited bacterial growth will occur around the disk.

A laboratory report (S & R report) can then be given to aid the clinician in choosing an antibiotic effective against the bacteria causing a particular infection. If the bacteria is not known, or cannot be cultured, or if time and the patient's health do not permit culturing and sensitivity studies prior to treatment, a broad-spectrum antibiotic may be employed to begin rapid treatment of infection.

**Fig 10–1.**—Illustration of a test dish of organisms, with inhibition of growth around two disks.

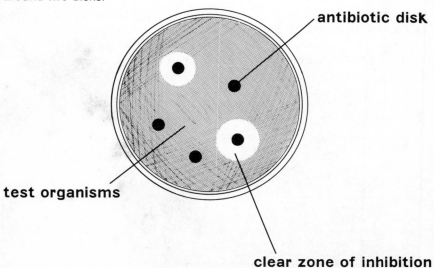

A disturbing aspect of the use of antibiotics is the development of bacterial strains which are resistant to particular antibiotics. The following example, which is qualitative, and not meant to represent actual data, can clarify the potential of this problem. In a colony of *Staphylococcus,* most individual bacteria may originally be vulnerable to an antibiotic such as penicillin. Perhaps 1% of the colony, however, is resistant, through genetic variations, to penicillin. The penicillin will effectively quell the infecting colony, by inhibiting growth in 99% of the bacteria; the number of organisms is reduced to a safe level; and the infected host will clear of symptoms (fever, inflammation, etc.). Nonetheless, the remaining 1% of bacteria will continue to grow and reproduce, so that ultimately an essentially new population of bacteria exists which is resistant to the penicillin. This antibiotic is no longer effective against the mutant strain of *Staphylococcus.* In reality, this has occurred in the clinical use of antibiotics. The more widespread and indiscreet the use of antibiotics, the more rapid the development of resistant, mutant strains is likely to be. The search for new, powerful antibiotics must keep pace with the growth of resistant strains which make currently effective antibiotics obsolete. For this reason too, antibiotic therapy is instituted in patients only when specifically indicated. It is not considered useful to chronic lung patients, to maintain them on continual antibiotic therapy, since the patient may acquire infection with resistant strains of bacteria. Generally, antibiotics are used at the first sign of infection with chronic obstructive lung patients.

## AEROSOLIZED ANTIBIOTICS IN RESPIRATORY CARE

Delivery of antibiotics by the inhalation route of administration using aerosolization of the drugs has been considered for pulmonary infections. The situation here is analogous to that with aerosolized corticosteroids: Can the tracheobronchial tree be treated *locally* without systemic levels of the drug resulting and causing harmful side effects?

It has been found that potentially toxic antibiotics can be delivered by aerosol to affect airway surfaces, with reduced systemic absorption.

The situation with pulmonary infections seems to be reducible to two general statements. First, the majority of pulmonary infections can be treated safely and effectively with oral or parenteral administration of antibiotics. Second, there is interest in the use of aerosolized antibiotics in the particular cases of resistant, colonizing, gram-negative pulmonary infections (e.g., *Pseudomonas*) and fungal infections protected within cavitary lesions, such as pulmonary aspergilloma or coccidioidomycosis.

1. GRAM-NEGATIVE PULMONARY INFECTIONS: Past reports (see reference list) have shown that the bacterial content of sputum can be altered with aerosolized antibiotics, but good clinical evidence is yet lacking that addition of aerosol antibiotics is actually superior therapeutically to systemic treatment alone. It has not been suggested that aerosol treatment *alone* be substituted for systemic treatment. A carefully controlled clinical trial of systemic antibiotic therapy versus systemic and aerosol therapy would be helpful to supply data here. Besides sputum bacterial content, other variables such as sputum volume, composition, viscosity and antibiotic systemic levels, as well as pulmonary status and diagnosis, would all need to be recorded.

   With regard to specific antibiotics, it has been found that kanamycin by aerosol (250 mg in 3 ml saline) will give a high lung tissue level with poor systemic absorption. Hazardous effects of auditory or renal damage are avoided. The effect on ventilatory mechanics with kanamycin is mild, whereas polymyxin (5–10 mg in 3 ml saline) by aerosol produced reductions in vital capacity and flow rates. If polymyxin is used by aerosol, a bronchodilator additive to prevent bronchospasm is indicated. Of the two agents, kanamycin offers promise for future investigation with pulmonary infections. Since antibiotics can be inactivated by combination with the DNA strands found in infected sputum, addition of a proteolytic enzyme, such as dornase, was considered. The enzyme broke down the DNA content of the sputum, to preserve the activity of the antibiotic, and also lower the viscosity of the secretions (see Chapter 6).

2. CAVITARY FUNGAL LESIONS: Treatment of fungal infections growing within the walls of a cavity is peculiarly difficult by systemic routes. Use of antibiotics in aerosol form, or by direct instillation through an endobronchial catheter, has given improvement and radiographic clearing. This was noted with use of amphotericin B in cases of pulmonary aspergillosis. As with gram-negative infections, further clinical evaluations in controlled studies are needed.

The hazards of the use of antibiotics by aerosol must be considered, as with any route of drug administration. They include bronchospasm, opportunistic infection, and sensitivity to the antibiotic with allergic reaction. An additional hazard, which respiratory care personnel should be aware of, is the potential legal implication with an adverse patient reaction, since the aerosol route of administration is not traditional for antibiotic therapy. Clear and specific physician orders are a minimal necessity for such a method, because of its somewhat experimental nature. In addition, hospital policy on such a use should be stated, and consultation with a department medical director should be required.

## REFERENCES

Adelson, H. T., and Malcolm, J. A.: Endocavitary treatment of pulmonary mycetomas, Am. Rev. Respir. Dis. 98:87, 1968.

Dickie, K. J., and de Groot, W. J.: Ventilatory effects of aerosolized kanamycin and polymyxin, Chest 63:694, 1973.

Greenfield, S., et al.: Prevention of gram-negative bacillary pneumonia using aerosol polymyxin as prophylaxis, J. Clin. Invest. 52:2935, 1973.

Ikemoto, H.: Treatment of pulmonary aspergilloma with amphotericin B, Arch. Intern. Med. 115:598, 1965.

Johanson, W. B., et al.: Nosocomial respiratory infections with gram-negative bacilli. The significance of colonization of the respiratory tract, Ann. Intern. Med. 77:701, 1972.

Kilburn, K. H.: The innocuousness and possible therapeutic use of aerosol amphotericin B, Am. Rev. Respir. Dis. 80:441, 1959.

Lifschitz, M. I., and Denning, C. R.: Safety of kanamycin aerosol, Clin. Pharmacol. Ther. 12:91, 1971.

Ramirez, J.: Pulmonary aspergilloma endobronchial treatment, N. Engl. J. Med. 271:1281, 1964.

Waksman, S. A.: Antibiotics today, Bull. N.Y. Acad. Med. 42:623, 1966.

Williams, M. H., Jr.: Steroid and antibiotic aerosols, Am. Rev. Respir. Dis. 110:122, 1974.

CHAPTER **11**

# Skeletal Muscle Relaxants (Neuromuscular Blocking Agents)

THE CLASS OF DRUGS known as neuromuscular blocking agents has a long and fascinating history. Some of the most notable events in their development for modern clinical use indicate the wealth of interesting detail available. Curare is a generic name for a variety of closely related agents, almost all of which were originally used by South American Indians as arrow poisons. The paralyzing effect of curare on skeletal muscle insured capture even if the quarry was not killed outright by the arrow itself. Curare became known to Europeans soon after the discovery of the American continents, and late in the sixteenth century, actual samples of native preparations were taken to Europe by explorers.

Curare can be extracted from several plants, one of which is *Chondodendron tomentosum,* a source of *d*-tubocurarine. The structure of *d*-tubocurarine was elicited by King, and reported in 1935. The semisynthetic derivative of *d*-tubocurarine, dimethyl tubocurarine, is approximately three times as potent as *d*-tubocurarine.

Griffith and Johnson reported the first trial use of curare as a muscle relaxant in general anesthesia in 1942.

Further research on curare-like drugs led to the discovery of gallamine, reported in 1949, and to the methonium compounds (hexamethonium, a ganglionic blocker, and decamethonium [Syncurine], a neuromuscular blocker) in 1948 and 1949.

Another neuromuscular blocker with a mode of action different from that of curare, and of great clinical use for surgery today, is succinylcholine (Anectine, Quelicin). It is interesting that this drug was used experimentally as early as 1906, but since research workers used *curarized* animals for testing succinylcholine, the muscle relaxant abilities of succinylcholine were not noticed until nearly forty years later!

110

In general, all of the neuromuscular blocking agents act through competitive inhibition with acetylcholine at the neuromuscular receptor site, or through a depolarizing action. Each of these mechanisms, and their concomitant effects, can be understood in terms of myoneural function.

## PHYSIOLOGY OF THE MYONEURAL JUNCTION

One of the branches of the peripheral nervous system, the somatic, or skeletal muscle, controls striated muscle, as opposed to smooth muscle found in bronchioles, myocardium, or arterioles, which are under the influence of the autonomic branch (see Fig 3–1). Examples of skeletal muscle include the biceps, triceps, and diaphragm, and all are responsible for motor functions such as lifting, walking, and breathing. In addition, these motor functions are under conscious cerebral control, which is not true of autonomically controlled smooth muscle.

Nervous impulses to stimulate skeletal muscle are carried via the somatic neuron to the myoneural synapse. Here the terminal end of the neuron releases acetylcholine when the electrical impulse arrives; in turn, the acetylcholine diffuses across the synaptic cleft to reach receptor sites on the muscle sole plate. Attachment of the acetylcholine causes *depolarization* of the postsynaptic membrane, and contraction of the muscle. The enzyme acetylcholinesterase, contained in storage sites, then inactivates the acetylcholine, repolarization of the membrane occurs, and new stimulation is possible (Fig 11–1).

## NEUROMUSCULAR BLOCKERS

On the basis of the myoneural function just described, two avenues become apparent for interruption of normal nervous stimulation of skeletal muscles:

1. Blockade of the receptor sites usually reached by acetylcholine, through use of a drug similar in structure to acetylcholine.
2. Stimulation and prolonged depolarization of the postsynaptic receptors.

### Nondepolarizing Blockers

The first method describes the action of nondepolarizing agents, such as curare, which maintain the membrane in a hyperpolarized state. No stimulation or depolarization occurs with these drugs; there

## NEUROMUSCULAR SYNAPSE

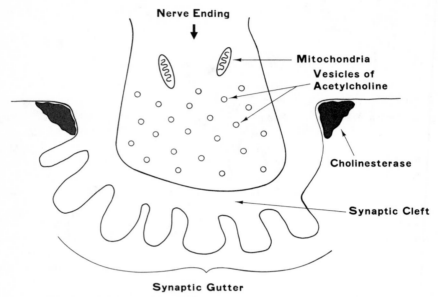

**Fig 11–1.**—Myoneural junction and neurotransmitter.

is simply blockade of the motor end-plate. IV injection of curare causes reaction within 1–2 minutes: haziness of vision, drooping eyelids, relaxation of the jaw, inability to raise the head, paralysis of the legs, arms, and, finally, loss of respiratory muscles ensues. Histamine release occurs as a side effect with symptoms of hypotension, bronchospasm, and exocrine gland secretion in evidence. The histamine release precipitated by curare can be reduced by use of synthetic derivatives such as pancuronium (Pavulon), which is particularly helpful in asthmatic patients. Antidotes to curare and other nondepolarizing drugs are parasympathomimetics such as edrophonium (Tensilon) or neostigmine (Prostigmin). These agents block the cholinesterase enzyme, and more acetylcholine is available to compete with the blocking curare and displace the curare from the receptor sites. Since they are parasympathomimetics, edrophonium and neostigmine also cause exocrine gland stimulation (lacrimal, bronchial, salivary), and atropine is usually given to offset this muscarinic effect. The atropine only blocks parasympathetic stimulation, not the skeletal muscle action of the two agents, to prevent accumulation of secretions in the patient's airway.

## Depolarizing Blockers

The basic action of depolarizing neuromuscular blockers is to fire, or depolarize, the postsynaptic membrane, and then maintain it in a refractory state. As with curare, further stimulation and contraction is not possible until the drug is metabolized. *Unlike* curare, there is an initial muscle contraction, referred to as fasciculation, a classic sign of depolarizing agents such as succinylcholine (Anectine, Quelicin). Normally, plasma cholinesterase will metabolize succinylcholine (a choline ester) within a few minutes. Generally, depolarizing blockers are shorter acting than curare and its analogues. Unfortunately, there are no effective antidotes to depolarizing agents. Use of parasympathomimetics here will result in even more prolonged depolarization, since the neuromuscular synapse is already being held in a depolarized state, and further stimulation will simply continue to cause depolarization, with no resumption of muscle activity.

SENSITIVITY TO SUCCINYLCHOLINE: There are two types of cholinesterase in the body: "true," or acetylcholinesterase, found at parasympathetic nerve synapses and postsynaptic neuromuscular sites; and "pseudo," or butyrylcholinesterase, found in plasma.

The pseudocholinesterase in the plasma plays no known metabolic function but it does catalyze the hydrolysis of succinylcholine; i.e., it metabolizes succinylcholine (a choline ester) to an inactive form. A certain number of individuals have an atypical plasma cholinesterase, and a few have none. In either case, such individuals will not rapidly hydrolize the depolarizing neuromuscular blocker within minutes as usual, but will require hours of supported ventilation because of the prolonged paralysis of the respiratory muscles. Laboratory tests are available to determine atypical cholinesterases.

In certain patients, a prolonged duration of action (1–4 hours instead of 2–4 minutes) occurs with succinylcholine that is *not* associated with inadequate plasma cholinesterase. In such cases, it has been theorized that a nondepolarizing block has occurred following the depolarizing block, possibly because of the first metabolic product of succinylcholine, which is succinylmonocholine. If this is the case, then a cholinesterase inhibitor should help offset this secondary block, and may further explain why such parasympathomimetics as neostigmine are occasionally helpful in reversing or antagonizing a prolonged depolarizing neuromuscular blockade.

## NONDEPOLARIZING NEUROMUSCULAR BLOCKING AGENTS

### *d*-Tubocurarine (tubocurarine chloride)

STRENGTH: injectable, 3 mg/ml (10 ml, 20 ml vials); 15 mg/ml (1 ml ampule).

DOSAGE: average dose, 6–9 mg IV.

MODE OF ACTION: Neuromuscular blockade is achieved through competitive inhibition of the drug with acetylcholine for receptor sites at the myoneural synapse. Depolarization (firing) of the muscle does *not* occur as the drug attaches to the receptor sites. As with other diamines, histamine release may be triggered, causing a fall in blood pressure, and causing bronchoconstriction, especially in asthmatic patients with hyperreactive airways. This can be noticed as a fall in compliance while "bagging" the patient.

Paralysis occurs rapidly with IV injection. In an average of 10 minutes the effect begins to diminish, and muscle tone may be resumed in 40 minutes following a single dose.

Curare does not affect the central nervous system, especially the higher cortical centers, and suitable anesthesia or analgesia is necessary when surgical procedures are anticipated. The nightmarish result of total paralysis with alert awareness of all sensory input could otherwise become a reality.

*d*-Tubocurarine is intensified by certain *antibiotics* (neomycin, streptomycin, polymyxin B, kanamycin, viomycin) and *acidosis.* The drug's effects are antagonized by anticholinesterase parasympathomimetics, alkalosis, and hypothermia.

HAZARDS: Apnea without assisted ventilation will result in death; histamine release can cause difficulty in ventilating the patient.

### Dimethyl tubocurarine chloride (Mecostrin)

STRENGTH: injectable, 1 mg/ml (10 ml vial).

DOSAGE: 2 mg IV.

MODE OF ACTION: nondepolarizing neuromuscular blockade, as with *d*-tubocurarine.

### Dimethyl tubocurarine iodide (Metubine)

STRENGTH: injectable, 1 and 2 mg/ml (20 ml vial).
DOSAGE: 2 mg IV.
MODE OF ACTION: nondepolarizing neuromuscular blockade, as with
*d*-tubocurarine. Both this drug and dimethyl tubocurarine chloride (just described) are considered to be more potent than
*d*-tubocurarine.

### Gallamine triethiodide (Flaxedil)

STRENGTH: injectable, 20 mg/ml (10 ml vial); 100 mg/ml (1 ml ampule).
DOSAGE: 80 mg IV.
MODE OF ACTION: Similar to *d*-tubocurarine, except that there is
parasympatholytic action at vagal sites, as well as voluntary motor
nerve endings, possibly producing tachycardia.
HAZARDS: Patients sensitive to iodine may have a hypersensitivity
reaction since the molecule contains iodine.

### Pancuronium (Pavulon)

STRENGTH: 2 mg/ml (2 and 5 ml ampules); 1 mg/ml (10 ml vial).
DOSAGE: 4–6 mg IV.
MODE OF ACTION: This drug is approximately 5 times as potent as
*d*-tubocurarine, and the basic mechanism is the same of neuromuscular blockade. However, the histamine release seen with
*d*-tubocurarine is largely absent, without the consequent symptoms of hypotension and bronchoconstriction.

## DEPOLARIZING NEUROMUSCULAR
## BLOCKING AGENTS

### Succinylcholine chloride (Anectine, Quelicin)

STRENGTH: 20, 50, and 100 mg/ml (10 ml vials).
DOSAGE: 30 mg IV.
MODE OF ACTION: After an initial depolarization of the myoneural
synapse with resulting fasciculation, the postsynaptic membrane
is held in a depolarized, refractory state, unable to be further
stimulated, and paralysis of the motor functions occurs. A fall in

blood pressure and bradycardia (parasympathomimetic effects) may be followed by a rise in arterial pressure and tachycardia because of a nicotinic effect (effect of acetylcholine on ganglionic and neuromuscular sites). Recall that succinylcholine has an affinity for receptors usually matched by acetylcholine, the neurotransmitter at the myoneural junction, as well as ganglionic and parasympathetic synapses. Paralysis is rapid with a short duration of action of 2–4 minutes unless a continuous IV drip is utilized. Good antidotes to depolarizing agents do not exist. The effect is intensified by antibiotics, hypothermia, or anticholinesterases.

HAZARDS: apnea, which is prolonged, with abnormal or missing plasma cholinesterases.

### Decamethonium (Syncurine)

STRENGTH: injectable, 1 mg/ml (10 ml vial).

DOSAGE: 2 MG IV.

MODE OF ACTION: depolarizing neuromuscular blockade. This drug is rarely used, and is largely being replaced by succinylcholine.

REFERENCES

Foldes, F. F.: The pharmacology of neuromuscular blocking agents in man, Clin. Pharmacol. Ther. 1:345, 1960.

Griffith, H. R., and Johnson, G. E.: The use of curare in general anesthesia, Anesthesiology 3:418, 1942.

Hunt, R., and Taveau, R. M.: On the physiological action of certain choline derivatives and new methods for detecting choline, Br. Med. J. 2:1788, 1906.

Katz, R. L.: Clinical neuromuscular pharmacology of pancuronium, Anesthesiology 34:550, 1971.

King, H.: Curare alkaloids. Part I. Tubocurarine, J. Chem. Soc. no. 330, p. 1381, 1935.

McIntyre, A. R.: *Curare: Its History, Nature, and Clinical Use* (Chicago: University of Chicago Press, 1947).

Rumble, L., et al.: Observations during apnea in conscious human subjects, Anesthesiology 18:419, 1957.

Taylor, D. B., and Nedergaard, O. A.: Relation between structure and action of quaternary ammonium neuromuscular blocking agents, Physiol. Rev. 45:523, 1965.

# CHAPTER 12

# Prostaglandins

IN 1934, Von Euler observed that seminal plasma possessed strong smooth muscle stimulating activity. The active substance responsible for this effect was later isolated and purified in the late 1950s and named prostaglandin. Prostaglandins are found in many parts of the body, not just in the testicular fluid. Since the 1950s there has been a dramatic increase in the interest in prostaglandin pharmacology and biochemistry in general, and within the last decade the importance of prostaglandins in relation to the lungs has become increasingly evident. In 1965, some 68 publications on prostaglandins appeared— twice the number previously existing. By 1972, publications neared two a day. The potential of prostaglandins for clinical and therapeutic use seems to be great at this point, and they may become a common clinical pharmacologic agent in the future. For that reason some understanding of the nature and function of prostaglandins in the pulmonary system is well indicated for respiratory care personnel.

## BASIC DESCRIPTION OF PROSTAGLANDINS

Prostaglandins are essentially 20-carbon, unsaturated fatty acids derived from a parent compound, prostanoic acid. The essential structure of the prostaglandin (PG) family is viewed in Figure 12–1. It is known that there are fourteen naturally occurring prostaglandins, which are divided into four groups: A, B, E, and F. The basic structure of all prostaglandins is a cyclopentane, or 5-atom ring, with two aliphatic side chains. A numerical subscript is added to the basic group letter, e.g., $E_2$, to refer to the number of unsaturated bonds in the aliphatic side chains. The three prostaglandins that are of greatest interest for pulmonary medicine are prostaglandin $E_1$, $E_2$, and $F_2\alpha$ (or $PGE_1$, $PGE_2$, and $PGF_2\alpha$). The basic difference between PGE and PGF lies in variations of the ring structure (Fig 12–2); however, the hydroxyl group at the carbon-15 site is essential for the ability of

117

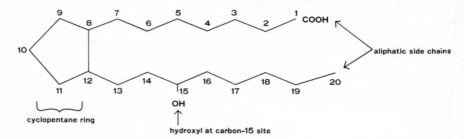

Basic Prostaglandin Structure

- 20-carbon unsaturated fatty acid.
- structure composed of cyclopentane ring (5-carbon ring) and 2 aliphatic side chains.
- hydroxyl at carbon-15 location essential for effects on smooth muscle.
- numerical subscripts, e.g. $PGE_1$, denote the number of double (unsaturated) bonds in the aliphatic side chains.
- Greek letters, e.g. $PGF_{2\alpha}$, indicate stereoisomeric forms.

**Fig 12–1.**—Key structural aspects and terminology of prostaglandins.

prostaglandins to alter smooth muscle tone. It is this pharmacologic effect that makes prostaglandins of potential benefit for respiratory care and airway maintenance. Within the human lung, $PGF_2\alpha$ has been found in the lung parenchyma and $PGE_2$, in the bronchi. To date, no $PGE_1$ or PGA has been found in human lung. It seems that most prostaglandin release in the lung involves synthesis following certain stimuli, rather than storage and release of the compound. In the circulation, prostaglandins have a very short half-life: 1–5 minutes for $PGF_2\alpha$. The vascular beds rapidly deactivate these compounds. In particular the pulmonary vascular bed is most effective with injected

**Fig 12–2.**—Classification of prostaglandins by major group, such as A, B, E, or F, is determined by the ring structure. The difference between PGE and PGF is shown.

configuration of ring determines major group (**A, B, E, F**)

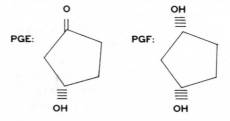

PGE and PGF metabolized in one passage through the lungs. The primary reaction in this deactivation involves first the oxidation of the crucial carbon-15 hydroxyl group by prostaglandin dehydrogenase, an enzyme which is found in great concentration in the lung. This initial reaction results in a loss of over 90% of the pharmacologic activity on smooth muscle by prostaglandin.

## Pharmacologic Effects

The crucial effect of prostaglandins in the lung is their ability to alter smooth muscle tone. There are two possible effects on smooth muscle, depending on the prostaglandin involved:

PGE—relaxation of bronchial smooth muscle

$PGF_2\alpha$—contraction of bronchial smooth muscle

Since these effects are not influenced by alpha- or beta-sympathetic agents, it seems that prostaglandins do not exert their effects through autonomic neurotransmitters or the autonomic pathway, nor do they attach to the same receptor sites that beta stimulants do. This is of extreme importance for respiratory care because the implication is that prostaglandins may offer an alternative pathway to affect smooth muscle tone, outside of the traditional autonomic pathways previously examined. Thus, for example, if a beta-sympathomimetic agent is ineffective, a prostaglandin may be a realistic alternative drug to utilize for smooth muscle relaxation.

Two additional factors favor the future importance of prostaglandins for respiratory care:

1. Prostaglandins are more potent by aerosol than by IV injection. This is related to the rapid deactivation in the pulmonary vascular bed, which occurs when the drug is introduced immediately into the bloodstream. Absorption in the respiratory mucosa does not cause this rapid deactivation.

2. Aerosolized PGE may have a potency greater than that of isoproterenol as a bronchodilator with asthmatic subjects. In conjunction with this, it is also noted that inhaled $PGF_2\alpha$ is more likely to induce bronchoconstriction in asthmatics than in normal subjects.

## Mode of Action

Evidence suggests that prostaglandins act directly on smooth muscle, and not through neural control or mediator release. Specifically, PGE exerts bronchodilation by stimulation of adenyl cyclase, causing

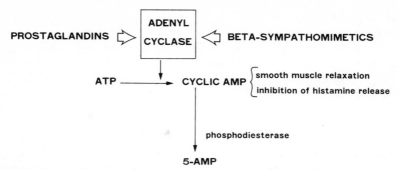

**Fig 12–3.**—Pathway by which prostaglandins increase cyclic AMP levels. Beta blockage does not inhibit PGE-induced rises in AMP.

an increase in cyclic AMP within the cell (Fig 12–3). This increase in cyclic AMP is not affected by beta-sympathomimetic blockers or beta blockade in asthmatics. It is this evidence that indicates that stimulation of adenyl cyclase is not through the autonomic neural pathway.

The effect of PGF is not well understood. It is suggested that the PGF effect is mediated via the cyclic GMP system, since cyclic GMP is thought to produce opposite effects of cyclic AMP (see Chapters 3 and 5). It has been noted that aspirin and indomethacin, both anti-inflammatory agents, inhibit the synthesis and release of prostaglandins. Inhibition of $PGE_2$ in the lung may lead to bronchoconstriction, thus implicating prostaglandins in the mechanism of aspirin-sensitive asthmatics.

## CLINICAL ASPECTS OF PROSTAGLANDINS

Prostaglandin release is associated with each of the following clinical situations:

1. Anaphylaxis—PGE and PGF have been shown to be released in anaphylaxis, although the extent to which these agents contribute to the processes of anaphylaxis is unknown.
2. Mechanical stimulation—Mechanical stretching of the lung provokes PG synthesis and release. This may be mainly of the PGE type, which then would be a cause of the hypotension associated with positive pressure and high lung inflation, formerly thought to be due only to impeded venous return and loss of thoracic pump. Certain anti-inflammatory agents such as aspirin or indomethacin are known to prevent the synthesis and release of prostaglandins by the lung. In studies with dogs,

pretreatment with aspirin, followed by progressive hyperinflation of the lungs, prevented up to 40% of the hypotension. Thus it is evident that a large part of the hypotension seen with large ventilation volumes, or positive end-expiratory pressure (PEEP), may be due to prostaglandins.

3. Hyperventilation—A low $PCO_2$ may be another stimulus to PG release in the lung.

4. Pulmonary embolism—Acute pulmonary embolism usually is associated with bronchoconstriction and systemic hypotension. The bronchoconstriction may be due to the particulate embolization provoking release of PGF, whereas the systemic hypotension may be due to a sequence of kallikrein conversion of kininogens to bradykinin, one of the mediators of anaphylaxis. The lung is particularly rich in the kallikrein enzymes, and is a rich source of kinin.

5. Pulmonary edema—Pulmonary edema as well as hypoxic breathing have both been found to stimulate the production and release of prostaglandins.

Because of their effect on both bronchial smooth muscle as well as blood vessels, prostaglandins may well have an important role in regulating ventilation-perfusion balance in the lung. Several examples can be drawn to illustrate this possibility.

First, it is known that carbon dioxide is a vasoconstrictor in the lung although it is a systemic vasodilator, and oxygen is a vasodilator in the lung although a systemic vasoconstrictor. Therefore in hyperventilation (see 3), PGE synthesis and release could relax pulmonary blood vessels, to induce vasodilation and increase perfusion. This may be the mediating or cooperating mechanism by which low $CO_2$ or high oxygen causes vasodilation in the lung.

Second, and by contrast, hypoxia may produce pulmonary vasoconstriction by the opposite effect through the mediation of PGF, which would produce vasoconstriction.

The lung seems to be particularly active both in the synthesis, as well as the metabolism, of prostaglandins, and with the effects of prostaglandins indicated by early research, these agents may become essential in respiratory care. Many aspects, especially of therapeutic clinical use, are not known, and no attempt is made to explain all pulmonary effects with these new substances. It is more likely that a complex situation of interacting mediators both cooperating and antagonizing each other exists in the lung. Some of the questions relating to this issue would be: Which situations produce which prostaglandins—i.e., what situation will produce PGE and therefore bronchodilation and vasodilation? Or which situation will produce PGF and bronchoconstriction/vasoconstriction? What factors affect the site of the prostaglandin release—i.e., are they released primarily in the bronchi, the parenchyma, or in the blood vessels of the lung? Research to answer these questions, and thereby to produce new pharmacologic agents for pulmonary treatment is being pursued by some of the major American drug companies at this time. We may well see these agents in our arsenal of respiratory care drugs in the future.

## REFERENCES

Bergstrom, S., Carlson, L. A., and Weeks, J. R.: The prostaglandins: A family of biologically active lipids, Pharmacol. Rev. 20:1, 1968.

Cuthbert, M. F.: Effect on airways resistance of prostaglandin $E_1$ given by aerosol to healthy and asthmatic volunteers, Br. Med. J. 4:723, 1969.

Euler, U. S. von: A depressor substance in the vesicular gland, J. Physiol. (Lond.) 84:21P, 1935.

Giraldo, B., Blumenthal, M. N., and Spink, W. W.: Aspirin intolerance and asthma, Ann. Intern. Med. 71:479, 1969.

Nakano, J., and Koss, M. C.: Pathophysiologic roles of prostaglandins and the action of aspirin-like drugs, South. Med. J. 66:709, 1973.

Parker, C. W., and Snider, D. E.: Prostaglandins and asthma, Ann. Intern. Med. 78:963, 1973.

Penna, P. M.: Bronchial asthma induced by aspirin and other analgesics: Review of incidence, mechanisms, and predisposing factors, Respir. Care 21:1135, 1976.

Said, S. I.: The lung in relation to vasoactive hormones, Fed. Proc. 32:1972, 1973.

Said, S. I., and Yoshida, T.: Release of prostaglandins and other humoral mediators during hypoxic breathing and pulmonary edema, Chest (suppl.) 66:12S, 1974.

Samter, M., and Beers, R. F.: Concerning the nature of intolerance to aspirin, J. Allergy 40:281, 1967.

Samter, M., and Beers, R. F.: Intolerance to aspirin. Clinical studies and consideration of its pathogenesis, Ann. Intern. Med. 68:975, 1968.

Shaw, J. O., and Moser, K. M.: The current status of prostaglandins and the lungs, Chest 68:75, 1975.

Smith, A. P., and Cuthbert, M. F.: Antagonistic action of aerosols of prostaglandins $F_2\alpha$ and $E_2$ in bronchial muscle tone in man, Br. Med. J. 3:212, 1972.

# CHAPTER 13

# Systems of Drug Distribution in Respiratory Therapy

IN RESPIRATORY THERAPY TODAY, the bulk of drug usage is in aerosol therapy, most of which is delivered with intermittent positive-pressure breathing (IPPB) machines. Throughout different institutions, a variety of methods exists for drawing up and measuring out drug dosages. While a definitively complete listing of methods used is not possible, nor even useful, certain major systems may be identified. Each of these systems is considered as a means of mixing together an *active ingredient,* such as isoproterenol, with a *diluent solution,* such as normal saline or distilled water. This situation of combining measured diluent and active ingredient is the most problematic for drug distribution in respiratory therapy. Any situation requiring only one agent is obviously satisfied by one syringe drawing up the needed amount. With this general perspective, the following systems can be discussed as alternative methods for measuring and mixing an active ingredient with a diluting agent.

## SEPARATE-SYRINGE METHOD

In the separate-syringe method, one syringe contains diluent, such as saline or water, and a second, separate syringe is used to draw up the prescribed amount of active ingredient. This method is most effective when an active ingredient, such as isoproterenol or acetylcysteine, is to be diluted in a second substance. The method is especially accurate if a syringe with fine gradations, e.g., a tuberculin syringe, is used when small amounts of a drug are required. This would be the case when 4 drops (or ¼ ml) of Bronkosol or another potent drug are needed.

DISADVANTAGES: mainly practical ones. If a large number of medications must be prepared and carried, a potentially large number of syringes will need to be prepared and carried. There is time-consuming labelling of numerous syringes, with duplication of patient name and location, and medication errors can result because of the number of syringes to be carried.

ADVANTAGES: the prevention of cross-contamination between diluent and active ingredient containers, and the accuracy of tuberculin or similar syringes. Droppers are provided with certain drugs, such as acetylcysteine and Bronkosol, but unless a dropper is *specifically* calibrated to a particular drug, it may be inaccurate. All drops are not created equally by differing droppers!

## SINGLE-SYRINGE METHOD

An alternative to two syringes is the practice of using one syringe to draw up both diluent and active ingredient. Usually the diluent is drawn from a multidose vial of saline or water, and then the additional amount of the second agent (usually a bronchodilator) is drawn up.

DISADVANTAGES: cross-contamination and possibly dilution of the second drug container (vial, bottle), as well as inaccuracy in the amount of the second ingredient, which must be visualized in a partially filled syringe.

ADVANTAGES: A reduction in the number of syringes prepared and carried is an advantage, but this convenience does not outweigh the potential hazards of the poor technique when more than one agent is needed. The single syringe is certainly suitable if only *one* agent is required.

## OPEN-CUP METHOD

The open-cup method utilizes small, 30 ml plastic medication cups, in which measured amounts of drugs are added and mixed, using syringes, or syringe and dropper. The resulting mixture can then be drawn back up by a single syringe.

DISADVANTAGES: contamination of drugs by nonsterile mixing containers and ambient conditions, and possible loss of small amounts of drugs.

ONE ADVANTAGE: Cross-contamination between vials can possibly be prevented if separate syringes are used to draw up diluent and active agent. There is also the convenience of having the final drug solution in one syringe. Of course, use of the cup for mixing implies more than one agent is needed. Otherwise the single syringe would be sufficient.

## UNIT-DOSE METHOD

A single unit-dose consists of exactly one dose of a drug or drugs apportioned in an individual dispenser. These unit-doses may be prepared by a commercial manufacturer in the same manner as prepared-strength capsules and tablets; by a hospital pharmacy; or by the respiratory therapy department itself, according to a suitable protocol. If the department or pharmacy prepares unit-dose medications, they may use a technique based on sound aseptic methods, or the suggested elements of a procedure described here. The crucial distinguishing feature of this method is that of systematic, uniform preparation of all medications by one or several persons, for use by the individual staff as they administer treatments. In essence, a *system,* and a *single-delivery vehicle,* is contrasted with multiple-dose or other forms drawn up in random fashion by all personnel operating individually.

DISADVANTAGES: a slight lack of flexibility in meeting unusual or unanticipated emergency drug dosages, and possibly a greater cost, depending on the exact system developed. Both of these disadvantages are most often encountered with commercially prepared unit-dose systems. A backup method of drawing up and mixing medications by the general staff must be available to handle situations of a "prn" nature, or when the usual medication staff is not present—if that should occur. Cost need not be a disadvantage if an in-hospital system of preparation is developed. The same supplies, and little extra manpower, would suffice as with any of the other methods in practice today.

ADVANTAGES: precision, accuracy, efficiency, and quality control in preparing and labelling patient drug doses. Assuming good technique (specified next) in preparing the medication, the unit-dose method is considered a superior form of drug delivery—and the preferred method.

## GENERAL SUGGESTIONS FOR DRUG PREPARATION IN RESPIRATORY THERAPY

MEASURING MEDICATIONS: Use one separate syringe for each drug agent or diluent; use tuberculin syringes for measuring potent bronchodilators or drugs with small, critical amounts. Add the measured drug or drugs, and diluent if needed, to a 3 ml syringe through the needle adapter on the syringe barrel; this 3 ml syringe will be the delivery vehicle for an actual unit-dose. After the delivery syringe or other suitable delivery container is filled, it can be capped and labelled with the medication name, dosage, date, patient's name, and location. A convenient label is the press-apply type of strip. This gives a unit-dose container, and, as a method of drug measurement, can be employed within a fully developed unit-dose drug preparation system, or by individual staff. The procedure is more efficient with one person drawing up a number of unit-syringes from the individual drug agents, rather than many staff members each drawing up a few doses. One medication technician would also better utilize a well-maintained work-space for preparing medications. An aseptic, established work-space for medication preparation, with all suitable supplies readily at hand, is a must for efficient operation.

CLARIFYING PHYSICIAN ORDERS: Check the physician's order for accuracy, and communicate to physicians the available drugs for aerosol use, and suggested strengths and dosages. This can be accomplished through the medical director or memoranda to the hospital's medical board.

MANUFACTURERS' SPECIFICATIONS: Check and follow all recommendations made by manufacturers concerning drug use. Valuable information is contained in drug literature inserts.

BASIC METHODOLOGY: A review of procedures should check for sound methods in all aspects of medication preparation. This includes basic handwashing, asepsis of the medication area and storage, labelling of drug doses, dating opened medications and discarding expired drugs, needle storage, and the overall process of drug distribution between the physician's order and actual administration of the drug to the patient. This process should be examined for streamlined efficiency and accuracy.

Because institutions differ in their needs and policies, a detailed, comprehensive, "ideal" drug procedure cannot be specified. Instead it is more profitable to offer a critical presentation of major methods of mixing and drawing up drugs, and then examine the elements of a procedure. These elements can be fitted together with whatever organizational skeleton is most suitable. For example, the system suggested here for measuring medications can be used by a hospital pharmacy preparing all drugs for a respiratory therapy department, or by a medication technician within the respiratory therapy department. The suggested procedures are nothing more than modules to be incorporated in whatever organizational structure works best for a given institution. In general, the unit-dose method, drawn up as described in these suggestions, is considered the method of choice.

## REFERENCES

Boyd, S.: Unit dose: A possible answer to contamination risk in IPPB nebulizer solutions, Respir. Care 18:428, 1973.

Griffin, B. T., and Batey, J. L.: Pharmacy-prepared unit-dose medications for respiratory therapy, Respir. Care 19:596, 1974.

Kohan, S., Carlin, H., and Whitehead, R.: A study of contamination of multiple-dose medication vials, Hospitals 36:14, 1962.

Mullen, A. F.: Dropper inaccurate for isoproterenol (letter), Respir. Care 20:619, 1975.

CHAPTER **14**

# Mathematics of Drug Dosage Calculation and Dosage Problems

The problems and exercises that follow are included for practice in the arithmetic of drug calculations and in actual drug dosage calculation. The arithmetic pretest covers the five basic areas of Roman numerals, fractions, decimals, proportions, and percentages. The arithmetic exercises are also divided into these five areas, to allow practice in any area or areas of difficulty. Drug dosage problems are provided, ranging from metric-apothecary conversions, to problems of solutions and percentage strengths, and calculating prepared-strength drug amounts.

### ARITHMETIC PRETEST

1. Write the arabic or Roman numeral equivalent.

   a. CLXIV = _____      f. 19 = _____

   b. VIII = _____      g. 43 = _____

   c. XVI = _____      h. 4 = _____

   d. XLI = _____      i. 67 = _____

   e. CXI = _____      j. 81 = _____

2. Change to whole numbers or to mixed numbers.

   a. $\frac{24}{12}$ = _____      c. $\frac{100}{25}$ = _____      e. $\frac{500}{25}$ = _____

   b. $\frac{9}{4}$ = _____      d. $\frac{16}{3}$ = _____      f. $\frac{67}{15}$ = _____

3. Add the following fractions.

   a. $\frac{1}{5} + \frac{1}{2} + \frac{1}{4}$ = _____

128

b. $\frac{1}{6} + \frac{3}{8} + \frac{3}{4} =$ _____

c. $2\frac{3}{4} + 4\frac{1}{8} + 5\frac{1}{2} =$ _____

4. Subtract the following fractions and mixed numbers.

   a. $\frac{2}{3} - \frac{1}{2} =$ _____     c. $4\frac{1}{2} - 2\frac{1}{3} =$ _____

   b. $\frac{4}{5} - \frac{1}{3} =$ _____     d. $10\frac{1}{4} - 6\frac{3}{8} =$ _____

5. Write as a decimal.

   a. forty-five and five-tenths = _____

   b. thirty-five and three-hundredths = _____

   c. two and five ten-thousandths = _____

   d. one hundred sixty and three-thousandths = _____

6. Add the following decimals.

   a. $0.05 + 0.010 + 0.156 =$ _____

   b. $1.005 + 20.1 + 400.5 =$ _____

   c. $0.004 + 42.015 + 1004.05 =$ _____

7. Subtract the following decimals.

   a. $12.05 - 10.50 =$ _____     c. $125.50 - 100.60 =$ _____
   b. $9.00 - 5.50 =$ _____     d. $95.05 - 5.25 =$ _____

8. Multiply the following.

   a. $525 \times 0.51 =$ _____     c. $594.99 \times 0.99 =$ _____

   b. $550.10 \times 0.05 =$ _____     d. $841.08 \times 0.08 =$ _____

9. Divide the following.

   a. $\frac{3}{5} \div \frac{3}{10} =$ _____     c. $14.25 \div 3.5 =$ _____
   b. $\frac{4}{8} \div \frac{1}{16} =$ _____     d. $150.25 \div .25 =$ _____

10. Change the following fractions to decimals.
    a. $\frac{7}{10} =$ _____     b. $5\frac{1}{4} =$ _____

11. Solve the following proportions.

    a. $1 : 2 :: X : 15$
    b. $30 : 45 :: 35 : X$          d. $\frac{17}{22} = \frac{34}{X}$

    c. $\frac{3}{4} = \frac{1}{X}$          e. $X : 60 :: 3 : 12$

12. Change the following to percentages.

　　a. $\frac{1}{2}$ = _____　　　　　c. $\frac{3}{4}$ = _____

　　b. 0.007 = _____　　　　d. 0.05 = _____

13. What is:

　　a. 5% of 75 = _____　　　　c. 6% of 400 = _____

　　b. 0.5% of 500 = _____　　　d. 0.7% of 750 = _____

### ANSWERS TO ARITHMETIC PRETEST

1. a. 164
   b. 8
   c. 16
   d. 41
   e. 111
   f. XIX
   g. XLIII
   h. IV
   i. LXVII
   j. LXXXI
2. a. 2
   b. $2\frac{1}{4}$
   c. 4
   d. $5\frac{1}{3}$
   e. 20
   f. $4\frac{7}{15}$
3. a. $\frac{19}{20}$
   b. $\frac{31}{24}$
   c. $\frac{99}{8}$

4. a. $\frac{1}{6}$
   b. $\frac{7}{15}$
   c. $\frac{13}{6}$
   d. $\frac{31}{8}$
5. a. 45.5
   b. 35.03
   c. 2.0005
   d. 160.003
6. a. 0.216
   b. 421.605
   c. 1046.069
7. a. 1.55
   b. 3.50
   c. 24.90
   d. 89.80
8. a. 267.75
   b. 27.505
   c. 589.0401
   d. 67.2864

9. a. $\frac{30}{15}$ = 2
   b. $\frac{64}{8}$ = 8
   c. 4.07
   d. 601
10. a. 0.7
    b. 5.25
11. a. 7.5
    b. 52.5
    c. $\frac{4}{3}$ or $1\frac{1}{3}$
    d. 44
    e. 15
12. a. 50%
    b. 0.7%
    c. 75%
    d. 5%
13. a. 3.75
    b. 2.5
    c. 24
    d. 5.25

## ARITHMETIC EXERCISES

Practice drills are offered in Roman numerals, fractions, decimals, ratios, and percentages. Rules and definitions are given first, with practice problems following. Answers may be found at the end of the section.

## Roman Numerals

Pharmacology uses both arabic (1, 2, 3 . . . ) and Roman numerals (i, ii, I, II). The following drill is designed to aid in becoming familiar with these symbols. Identification of symbols and rules of use are given first.

RULES:

| | |
|---|---|
| i, I = 1 | C = 100 |
| v, V = 5 | D = 500 |
| x, X = 10 | M = 1,000 |
| L = 50 | |

Reading from left to right, *add* amounts, placing largest numerals to left.

EXAMPLE: 27 is XXVII

If a smaller numeral is before (to the left of) a larger numeral, *subtract* the smaller from the larger.

EXAMPLE: 29 is XXIX

Use the shortest form of a number when more than one form is possible.

EXAMPLE: LLIV → CIV = 104
XIIII → XIV = 14

EXERCISE: Represent by Roman numerals.

a. 5 = _____          f. 100 = _____

b. 1 = _____          g. 105 = _____

c. 9 = _____          h. 95 = _____

d. 7 = _____          i. 596 = _____

e. 4 = _____          j. 16 = _____

EXERCISE 2: Interpret the following:

a. XV = _____          f. CXIII = _____

b. LXVII = _____          g. CMLXI = _____

c. MCMLXXVI = _____          h. XLIII = _____

d. XXI = _____          i. CDXXXVI = _____

e. VIII = _____          j. XXXIX = _____

EXERCISE 3: Additional problems.

a. 44 = _____          c. 942 = _____

b. 88 = _____          d. 1652 = _____

　　e. 409 = _____        h. 1847 = _____

　　f. 1966 = _____        i. 448 = _____

　　g. 2004 = _____        j. 3041 = _____

　　　　　　　　　　　　　　k. 709 = _____

EXERCISE 4: Easy problems.

　　a. 18 = _____        f. 73 = _____

　　b. 23 = _____        g. 13 = _____

　　c. 34 = _____        h. 42 = _____

　　d. 186 = _____        i. 324 = _____

　　e. 88 = _____        j. 2 = _____

### Fractions

#### TERMS

*Fraction:* a portion of a whole.

*Numerator:* upper number of fraction, which is the dividend.

*Denominator:* lower number of fraction, the divisor.

EXAMPLE: $\underline{2}$ (numerator)
　　　　　3 (denominator)

*Least common denominator (LCD:)* for a group of fractions, the *smallest* number that all of the denominators will divide into evenly.

EXAMPLE: for $\frac{1}{2}$ and $\frac{1}{3}$, LCD = 6 $\therefore \frac{1}{2} = \frac{3}{6}, \frac{1}{3} = \frac{2}{6}$

*Proper fraction:* numerator is *less than* denominator.

EXAMPLE: $\frac{4}{5}$

*Improper fraction:* numerator is *greater than* denominator.

EXAMPLE: $\frac{5}{4}$

*Complex fraction:* a fraction whose numerator, or denominator, or both, are fractions.

EXAMPLE: $\frac{1/2}{3}, \frac{1/2}{2/3}$

*Mixed number:* a whole number and a fraction.

EXAMPLE: $1\frac{2}{3}$

#### REDUCING FRACTIONS

RULE: To reduce fractions, find a number which divides evenly into both numerator and denominator.

**EXERCISE 5:** Reduce the following fractions.

a. $\frac{6}{24}$ = _____     f. $\frac{4}{16}$ = _____

b. $\frac{9}{27}$ = _____     g. $\frac{2}{7}$ = _____

c. $\frac{1}{3}$ = _____     h. $\frac{3}{4}$ = _____

d. $\frac{2}{8}$ = _____     i. $\frac{9}{16}$ = _____

e. $\frac{2}{4}$ = _____     j. $\frac{4}{24}$ = _____

**EXERCISE 6:** Find the least common denominator.

a. $\frac{3}{4}$ , $\frac{1}{6}$ , $\frac{1}{2}$ : LCD = _____     f. $\frac{1}{24}$ , $\frac{3}{12}$ , $\frac{1}{4}$ : LCD = _____

b. $\frac{1}{18}$ , $\frac{1}{9}$ , $\frac{3}{18}$ : LCD = _____     g. $\frac{1}{24}$ , $\frac{5}{6}$ , $\frac{1}{48}$ : LCD = _____

c. $\frac{3}{4}$ , $\frac{3}{12}$ , $\frac{4}{9}$ : LCD = _____     h. $\frac{9}{27}$ , $\frac{2}{3}$ , $\frac{1}{8}$ : LCD = _____

d. $\frac{3}{20}$ , $\frac{1}{9}$ , $\frac{3}{18}$ : LCD = _____     i. $\frac{6}{13}$ , $\frac{1}{26}$ , $\frac{5}{6}$ : LCD = _____

e. $\frac{7}{20}$ , $\frac{5}{8}$ : LCD = _____     j. $\frac{6}{18}$ , $\frac{3}{6}$ , $\frac{1}{2}$ : LCD = _____

## MIXED NUMBERS AND IMPROPER FRACTIONS

**RULES:** To change mixed numbers to improper fractions:
1. Multiply the whole number by the fraction's denominator.
2. Add this product to the numerator.
3. The denominator stays the same.

**EXAMPLE:** $1\frac{2}{3} = \frac{3+2}{3} = \frac{5}{3}$

**RULES:** To change improper fractions to mixed numbers:
1. Divide the denominator into the numerator.
2. Write the remainder as a fraction, with the original denominator.

**EXERCISE 7:** Change to mixed numbers and improper fractions.

a. $1\frac{1}{4}$ = _____     g. $13\frac{1}{2}$ = _____

b. $1\frac{2}{3}$ = _____     h. $7\frac{7}{8}$ = _____

c. $4\frac{1}{8}$ = _____     i. $1\frac{3}{7}$ = _____

d. $1\frac{4}{6}$ = _____     j. $2\frac{1}{6}$ = _____

e. $3\frac{2}{5}$ = _____     k. $\frac{42}{7}$ = _____

f. $4\frac{2}{3}$ = _____     l. $\frac{56}{8}$ = _____

m. $\frac{9}{6}$ = _____   q. $\frac{13}{3}$ = _____

n. $\frac{8}{7}$ = _____   r. $\frac{16}{4}$ = _____

o. $\frac{19}{5}$ = _____   s. $\frac{7}{2}$ = _____

p. $\frac{43}{12}$ = _____   t. $\frac{16}{7}$ = _____

## ADDITION

RULES: Find a common denominator, then add the numerators together. Reduce improper fractions to mixed numbers. Reduce fractions whenever possible after adding.

EXERCISE 8: Add the following fractions, and reduce improper fractions to mixed numbers.

a. $\frac{3}{4} + \frac{1}{4}$ = _____   f. $\frac{1}{2} + \frac{7}{12}$ = _____

b. $\frac{2}{3} + \frac{1}{3}$ = _____   g. $\frac{3}{4} + \frac{1}{8}$ = _____

c. $\frac{3}{4} + \frac{1}{2}$ = _____   h. $\frac{2}{7} + \frac{1}{8}$ = _____

d. $\frac{1}{2} + \frac{4}{6}$ = _____   i. $\frac{5}{6} + \frac{1}{7}$ = _____

e. $\frac{2}{3} + \frac{3}{4}$ = _____   j. $\frac{6}{8} + \frac{2}{4}$ = _____

## MULTIPLICATION AND DIVISION

RULES: For multiplication:
1. Change any mixed numbers to improper fractions.
2. Cancel wherever possible.
3. Multiply remaining numerators to get final numerator, and remaining denominators to get denominator.

EXAMPLE: $1\frac{3}{5} \times \frac{2}{8}$ = ?
$\frac{8}{5} \times \frac{2}{8} = \frac{2}{5}$

RULE: For division:
1. Follow Rule 1 for multiplication.
2. Invert the divisor (fraction after division sign) and then multiply. Follow rules of multiplication.

EXERCISE 9: Multiply or divide these fractions.

a. $\frac{1}{2} \times \frac{3}{4}$ = _____   d. $\frac{1}{2} \times \frac{3}{8}$ = _____

b. $2\frac{1}{7} \times \frac{3}{21}$ = _____   e. $\frac{3}{8} \times 4\frac{1}{2}$ = _____

c. $\frac{6}{18} \times 1\frac{3}{6}$ = _____   f. $\frac{4}{12} \times \frac{1}{3}$ = _____

g. $\frac{3}{16} \times 2 =$ _____

h. $\frac{12}{24} \times \frac{3}{4} =$ _____

i. $\frac{1}{2} \div \frac{3}{16} =$ _____

j. $\frac{1}{2} \div 1\frac{1}{6} =$ _____

k. $4\frac{1}{2} \div \frac{1}{2} =$ _____

l. $6 \div \frac{2}{3} =$ _____

m. $2\frac{1}{4} \div \frac{1}{8} =$ _____

n. $\frac{2}{3} \div \frac{1}{3} =$ _____

o. $\frac{1}{2} \div 3 =$ _____

## Decimals

Decimals are based on tens, and multiples or fractions of ten. Reading decimals is as follows:

| t | t | h | t | u | t | h | t | t |
|---|---|---|---|---|---|---|---|---|
| e | h | u | e | n | e | u | h | e |
| n | o | n | n | i | n | n | o | n |
|   | u | d | s | t | t | d | u |   |
| t | s | r |   | s | h | r | s | t |
| h | a | e |   |   | s | e | a | h |
| o | n | d |   |   |   | d | n | o |
| u | d | s |   |   |   | t | d | u |
| s | s |   |   |   |   | h | t | s |
| a |   |   |   |   |   | s | h | a |
| n |   |   |   |   |   |   | s | n |
| d |   |   |   |   |   |   |   | d |
| s |   |   |   |   |   |   |   | t |
|   |   |   |   |   |   |   |   | h |
|   |   |   |   |   |   |   |   | s |

EXAMPLE: 0.29 is "twenty-nine hundreths"

1.2 is "one and two-tenths"

### ADDITION AND SUBTRACTION

RULE: For addition or subtraction, line up all decimals in a column, with the decimal points of all numbers in the same line.

EXAMPLE: 0.04

$\underline{+1.3}$

1.34

EXERCISE 10: Add or subtract.

a. $27.1 + 3.007 =$ _____

b. $127 + 0.1 =$ _____

c. $3.4 + 1 =$ _____

d. $6.9 + 1.745 =$ _____

e. $10.9 + 0.0075 =$ _____

f. $27.9 - 0.3 =$ _____

g. $375.4 - 1.7542 =$ _____

h. $10 - 0.001 =$ _____

i. $9.5 - 0.3 =$ _____

j. $675.2 - 3 =$ _____

## MULTIPLICATION

RULE: To multiply decimals:
1. Multiply as with whole numbers.
2. Count off the *total* number of decimal places in the figures multiplied from the right (to left) in your answer.

EXAMPLE: $0.23 \times 1.01 = 0.2323$

EXERCISE 11: Multiply.

a. $3.1 \times 1.75 =$ _____

b. $10 \times 0.1 =$ _____

c. $6.97 \times 1.34 =$ _____

d. $6 \times 0.003 =$ _____

e. $125 \times 1.0 =$ _____

f. $10 \times 0.9 =$ _____

g. $3.10 \times 2 =$ _____

h. $3.3 \times 11 =$ _____

i. $4.6 \times 2.3 =$ _____

j. $5.91 \times 3.1 =$ _____

## DIVISION

RULE: To divide decimals convert the divisor to a whole number (no decimals in it) if necessary, and move the decimal place in the dividend the same number of places to the *right*.

EXAMPLE: $0.18 \div 1.3$ becomes
$1.8 \div 13$

EXERCISE 12: Divide.

a. $10.3 \div 14.13 =$ _____

b. $193 \div 0.2 =$ _____

c. $0.13 \div 15.1 =$ _____

d. $12,400 \div 0.19 =$ _____

e. $87.6 \div 93.45 =$ _____

f. $1 \div 16 =$ _____

g. $1 \div 375 =$ _____

h. $2.478 \div 2.43 =$ _____

i. $76.648 \div 0.04 =$ _____

j. $3.0 \div 2.0 =$ _____

## Ratios

Ratios are commonly expressed in two formats:
As fractions: $\frac{1}{2} = \frac{2}{4}$

As proportional terms: 1 : 2 :: 2 : 4
extreme : means :: means : extreme
RULE: To solve ratios as fractions, cross-multiply the numerators with opposite denominator.
RULE: To solve ratios as proportions, mutiply the extremes, which will then equal the result of multiplying the means.
In the example just given this is:
$$1 \times 4 = 2 \times 2$$
If any one of the means or extremes is unknown, it can be called $X$, and then solved for:
$$1 \times 4 = 2 \times X$$
$$2X = 4$$
$$X = \tfrac{4}{2} = 2$$

EXERCISE 13: Solve the proportions or fractions.

a. 1 : 3 :: $X$ : 5

b. 0.02 : $X$ :: 101 : 43

c. $X$ : 55 :: 0.75 : 4.5

d. $\dfrac{12.2}{X} = \dfrac{1.1}{150}$

e. $\dfrac{X - 3}{5} = \dfrac{8}{10}$

f. $\dfrac{X}{46} = \dfrac{0.002}{0.47}$

g. $\dfrac{0.13}{1.8} = \dfrac{9}{X}$

h. $\dfrac{7}{13} = \dfrac{X}{65}$

i. 1 : 4 :: $X$ : 35

j. 1.5 : 2.35 :: 5 : $X$

## Percentages

*Percentage:* parts per hundred.
25% is 25 parts per hundred.
In decimals, this would be 0.25, or twenty-five hundredths.
In fractions: $\tfrac{25}{100}$
RULE: To express a percentage as a decimal *divide* by a hundred, which is to move the decimal two places toward the *left*.
EXAMPLE: 15.5% = 0.155
RULE: To express a decimal as a percent, *multiply* by a hundred, which is to move the decimal two places toward the *right*. (For a fraction, divide the denominator into the numerator to obtain a decimal.)
EXAMPLE: 0.364 = 36.4%
EXERCISE 14: Express as a decimal.

a. 47% = _____

b. 0.2% = _____

c. 50% = _____

d. 150% = _____

e. 15% = _____    g. 0.1% = _____

f. 36% = _____    h. 0.005% = _____

**EXERCISE 15:** Express as a percentage.

a. 0.5 = _____    f. 1/200 = _____

b. 0.125 = _____    g. 1/50 = _____

c. 0.56 = _____    h. 1/1000 = _____

d. 0.3 = _____    i. 1/100 = _____

e. 0.95 = _____

## ANSWERS TO ARITHMETIC EXERCISES

1. a. V
   b. I
   c. IX
   d. VII
   e. IV
   f. C
   g. CV
   h. XCV
   i. DXCVI
   j. XVI
2. a. 15
   b. 67
   c. 1976
   d. 21
   e. 8
   f. 113
   g. 961
   h. 43
   i. 436
   j. 39
3. a. XLIV
   b. LXXXVIII
   c. CMXLII
   d. MDCLII
   e. CDIX
   f. MCMLXVI
   g. MMIV

   h. MDCCCXLVII
   i. CDXLVIII
   j. MMMXLI
   k. DCCIX
4. a. XVIII
   b. XXIII
   c. XXXIV
   d. CLXXXVI
   e. LXXXVIII
   f. LXXIII
   g. XIII
   h. XLII
   i. CCCXXIV
   j. II
5. a. $\frac{1}{4}$
   b. $\frac{1}{3}$
   c. $\frac{1}{3}$
   d. $\frac{1}{4}$
   e. $\frac{1}{2}$
   f. $\frac{1}{4}$
   g. $\frac{2}{7}$
   h. $\frac{3}{4}$
   i. $\frac{9}{16}$
   j. $\frac{1}{6}$
6. a. 12
   b. 36
   c. 36

   d. 180
   e. 40
   f. 24
   g. 48
   h. 216
   i. 78
   j. 18
7. a. $\frac{5}{4}$
   b. $\frac{5}{3}$
   c. $\frac{33}{8}$
   d. $\frac{10}{6}$
   e. $\frac{17}{5}$
   f. $\frac{14}{3}$
   g. $\frac{27}{2}$
   h. $\frac{63}{8}$
   i. $\frac{10}{7}$
   j. $\frac{13}{6}$
   k. 6
   l. 7
   m. $1\frac{1}{2}$
   n. $1\frac{1}{7}$
   o. $3\frac{4}{5}$
   p. $3\frac{7}{12}$
   q. $4\frac{1}{3}$
   r. 4
   s. $3\frac{1}{2}$
   t. $2\frac{2}{7}$

8. a. $\frac{4}{4} = 1$
   b. $\frac{3}{3} = 1$
   c. $\frac{5}{4} = 1\frac{1}{4}$
   d. $\frac{7}{6} = 1\frac{1}{6}$
   e. $\frac{17}{12} = 1\frac{5}{12}$
   f. $\frac{13}{12} = 1\frac{1}{12}$
   g. $\frac{7}{8}$
   h. $\frac{23}{56}$
   i. $\frac{41}{42}$
   j. $\frac{10}{8} = 1\frac{2}{8} = 1\frac{1}{4}$
9. a. $\frac{3}{8}$
   b. $\frac{45}{147}$
   c. $\frac{1}{2}$
   d. $\frac{3}{16}$
   e. $\frac{27}{16}$
   f. $\frac{4}{36} = \frac{1}{9}$
   g. $\frac{6}{16}$
   h. $\frac{3}{8}$
   i. $\frac{8}{3} = 2\frac{2}{3}$
   j. $\frac{3}{7}$
   k. $\frac{9}{1} = 9$
   l. 9
   m. 18
   n. 2
   o. $\frac{1}{6}$
10. a. 30.107
    b. 127.1
    c. 4.4

d. 8.645
e. 10.9075
f. 27.6
g. 373.6458
h. 9.999
i. 9.2
j. 672.2
11. a. 5.425
    b. 1.0
    c. 9.3398
    d. 0.018
    e. 125
    f. 9.0
    g. 6.20
    h. 36.3
    i. 10.58
    j. 18.321
12. a. 0.72894
    b. 965.0
    c. 0.00860
    d. 65,263.157
    e. 0.93739
    f. 0.0625
    g. 0.00266
    h. 1.01975
    i. 1916.20
    j. 1.5

13. a. $X = 1.667$
    b. $X = 0.0085$
    c. $X = 9.167$
    d. $X = 1663.636$
    e. $X = 7$
    f. $X = 0.196$
    g. $X = 124.615$
    h. $X = 35$
    i. $X = 8.75$
    j. $X = 7.83$
14. a. 0.47
    b. 0.002
    c. 0.5
    d. 1.50
    e. 0.15
    f. 0.36
    g. 0.001
    h. 0.00005
15. a. 50%
    b. 12.5%
    c. 56%
    d. 30%
    e. 95%
    f. 0.005 = 0.5%
    g. 0.02 = 2%
    h. 0.001 = 0.1%
    i. 0.01 = 1%

## DRUG DOSAGE PROBLEMS

### Conversion Calculation Problems

1. An ointment calls for 4 drams of procaine HCl. How many grams is this? 4 drams = _____ grams?

2. 7.5 minims = _____ milliliters?

3. 1/150 grain = _____ milligrams?

4. 1/2 fluid ounce (apoth) = _____ milliliters?

5. How many grains are contained in 0.3 grams?

6. 8 fluid ounces (apoth) = _____ milliliters?

7. 3.0 grams = _____ grains?

8. 135 pounds (avdp) = _____ kilograms?

9. 0.5 gram = _____ grains?

10. 3 kilograms = _____ pounds (avdp)?

11. 10 milliliters = _____ cc's?

12. 10 milliliters = _____ minims?

13. 10 milliliters = _____ drops (gtt)?

14. 1/4 cc = _____ drops?

15. 1/4 cc = _____ minims?

16. 8 gtt = _____ cc's?


## Examples of Problems On Solutions

EXAMPLE 1: How many milligrams of active ingredient are in 3 ml of a 2% solution of procaine HCl?

Use the percentage formula, pure strength ingredient:

$$\% = \frac{\text{solute}}{\text{total amount}}$$

Convert % to decimals and substitute the known values:

$$0.02 = \frac{X \text{ gm}}{3 \text{ ml}}$$

$$X = 0.06 \text{ grams}$$

In milligrams:

$$0.06 \text{ gm} \times 1{,}000 \text{ mg/gm} = 60 \text{ mg}$$

$$\text{Answer: 60 mg}$$

EXAMPLE 2: How much active ingredient do you need for 10 ml of 2% procaine? Assume pure strength ingredient.
The formula:

$$\% = \frac{\text{solute}}{\text{total amount}}$$

Substitute:

$$0.02 = \frac{X \text{ gm}}{10 \text{ ml}}$$

$$X = 0.2 \text{ gm}$$
$$= 200 \text{ mg}$$

Answer: 200 mg

EXAMPLE 3: What size dose of 1:200 isoproterenol will deliver 7.5 mg active ingredient?

Convert 7.5 mg to gm (*Always use grams or milliliters!*):

$$7.5 \text{ mg} = 0.0075 \text{ gm}$$

And convert 1:200 to %:

$$1:200 = 1 \text{ gm to } 200 \text{ ml or,}$$
$$0.5 \text{ gm}/100 \text{ ml} = 0.5\%$$

Substitute:

$$\% = \frac{\text{solute}}{\text{total amount}}$$

$$0.005 = \frac{0.0075 \text{ gm}}{X \text{ amount}}$$

$$X = \frac{0.0075}{0.05}$$

$$= 1.5 \text{ ml or cc}$$

Answer: 1.5 ml

EXAMPLE 4: Bronkosol contains isoetharine 1.0%; how much active ingredient is contained in a normal 4 drop dose?

Convert 4 drops to ml:

$$1 \text{ ml} = 16 \text{ drops}$$

$$4 \text{ drops} = \tfrac{4}{16} \text{ ml} = \tfrac{1}{4} \text{ ml} = 0.25 \text{ ml}$$

Substitute:

$$0.01 = \frac{X \text{ gm}}{0.25 \text{ ml}}$$

$$X = 0.0025 \text{ gm}$$

$$= 2.5 \text{ milligrams}$$

Answer: 2.5 mg

EXAMPLE 5: What percentage strength is 14 grams in 40 ml of solution?

Substitute:

$$X = \frac{14 \text{ gm}}{40 \text{ ml}}$$

$$X = 0.35 = 35\%$$

Answer: 35%

No conversions are necessary since all units are in grams or milliliters as required by the definition of percentage strength.

## Problems on Solutions

17. How many grams of calamine are needed to prepare 120 grams of an ointment containing 8% calamine?
18. 1 ml of active enzyme is found in 147 ml of Dornavac. What is the percentage strength of active enzyme?
19. If Valium contained 2% active ingredient, how many grams of the active ingredient would be needed to make 20 grams of Valium?
20. You have Isuprel 1:100. How many milliliters of Isuprel would be needed to contain 30 mg of active ingredient?
21. A dose of 0.4 ml of epinephrine HCl, 1:1000, is ordered. This dose contains how many milligrams of epinephrine HCl (the active ingredient)?
22. What is the percentage strength of a 1:4000 solution of copper sulfate?
23. The maximum dose of Isuprel that may be given by aerosol for a particular patient is 3 milligrams. The drug is available as a 1:200 solution. What is the maximal amount of solution (in milliliters) of isoproterenol that may be used?
24. The maximum recommended single dose of chloroprocaine HCl for regional block is 800 milligrams. How many milliliters of a 2% solution contains 850 milligrams of the local anesthetic?
25. How many grams of zinc stearate should be used to prepare one apothecary pound of an ointment containing 35% zinc stearate? (Note: 12 apoth ounces = 1 apoth pound)
26. Calculate the percentage of the sulfur in an ointment if one pound (avdp) of the ointment contains 30 grams of sulfur?

## Problems on Drug Dosage Calculation

27. A bottle is labelled Demerol (meperidine) 50 mg/cc. How many cc are needed to give a 125 mg dose?

28. Promazine HCl comes as 500 mg/10 ml. How many milliliters are needed to give 150 mg dose?
29. Hyaluronidase comes as 150 units/cc. How many cc for a 30 unit dose?
30. Morphine sulfate 0.25 milligram is ordered for an infant. You have 15 mg/ml. How much do you need?
31. You have a morphine sulfate vial with ¼ gr/cc. How many cc for a 10 milligram dose?
32. Diphenhydramine (Benadryl) elixir contains 12.5 mg of diphenhydramine HCl in each 5 ml of elixir. How many milligrams are there in a one-half-teaspoonful dose?
33. How many aspirin tablets 0.3 gm should be administered if a 10 gr dose is ordered?
34. A pediatric dose of oxytetracycline 100 mg is ordered. The dosage form is an oral suspension containing 125 mg/5 cc. How much of the suspension contains a 100 mg dose?
35. Ephedrine sulfate capsules ¾ gr are ordered. How many milligrams is this?
36. Ferrous sulfate elixir contains 220 mg of ferrous sulfate per 5 ml dose. How much exilir should be given for a 5 gr dose of ferrous sulfate?

## Answers to Drug Dosage Problems

1. 14.4 gm, if you use 4 drams = 240 gr, 1 gr = 60 mg.
   15 gm, based on 4 drams = ½ oz, 1 oz = 30 gm.
2. 0.5 ml
3. 0.4 mg
4. 15 ml
5. 5 gr
6. 240 ml
7. 45 gr
8. 61.36 kg
9. 7.5 gr based on 1 gm = 15 gr
   8.33 gr based on 0.5 gm = 500 mg, and 1 gr = 60 mg
10. 6.6 lb (avdp)
11. 10 cc
12. 150 minims
13. 160 gtt
14. 4 gtt
15. 3.75 minims or approximately 4 minims (1 gtt = 1 minim)

16. 0.5 cc
17. 9.6 gm
18. 0.68%
19. 0.4 gm
20. 3.0 ml
21. 0.4 mg
22. 0.025%
23. $\frac{3}{5}$ ml = 0.6 ml
24. 42.5 ml
25. 126 gm
26. 6.6%
27. 2.5 cc
28. 3 ml
29. 0.2 cc
30. 0.0167 ml
31. 0.67 cc
32. 6.25 mg
33. 2 tablets
34. 4 cc
35. 45 mg
36. 6.8 ml

# Index

## A

Aarane, 100–103
Abbreviations: used in prescriptions,
    19
Absorption: of drug, 9–11
Acetylcholine, 38
Acetylcysteine, 71–73
    action mechanism, 72
    dosage, 71
    pH and, 72
ACTH: diurnal variations in, 91
Additive, 8
Adrenal
    cortex, 84–85
        neurosecretory control of, 87–89
    -hypothalamic-pituitary axis, 89
    medulla, 84
Adrenergic, 43
Aerolone, 56
Aerosol(s)
    cartridge, gas-powered, 17
    mistometer, 15–16
        problems with, 59–60
    Sch 1000, 63–64
        dosage, 63
Aerosolized antibiotics, 107–109
Airway patency, 20
Albuterol, 58
Alcohol, 79–80
    dosage, 79
    ethyl, 79–80
Alevaire, 80
Allergic (see Asthma, allergic)
Alpha receptors, 40
Alpha stimulation, 45
Alpha sympatholytics, 47
Alupent, 57
Aminophylline, 65
AMP, cyclic, 45–46
    beta pathway of, 97
    control, pathways, 102
    physiological effects of, 97
    prostaglandins and, 120
    release, pathways, 102
Anaphylaxis: and prostaglandins, 120
Anectine, 115–116

Antagonism, 8
Antiadrenergic, 43
Antiasthmatic: cromolyn sodium as, 96–
    103
Antibiotics, 104–109
    action modes, 104–105
    aerosolized, 107–109
    bactericidal, 105
    bacteriostatic, 105
    broad-spectrum, 106
    clinical aspects of, 105–107
    definition, 104
    history of, 104
    inhibiting
        cell membrane function, 104–105
        cell wall synthesis, 104
        nucleic acid synthesis, 105
        protein synthesis, 105
    narrow-spectrum, 106
Antibody, 98
    cytophilic, 100
    formation, 98
Anticholinergic, 43
Antigen, 98
    -antibody reaction, 98
Apothecary system, 24–25
Arithmetic
    exercises, 130–139
    pretest, 128–130
Asbron G, 66
Asthma, allergic
    mediator release from mast cell in, 101
    physiology of, 96–100
Atomizer, 14
Atopy, 97
Atropine, 63
    dosage, 63
Autonomic
    control in lung, unified theory of,
        44–47
    effects
        in cardiopulmonary system, 43
        mediated through intracellular nu-
            cleotides, 46
    nervous system (see Nervous system,
        autonomic)
Avoirdupois system, 25

### B

Bactericidal antibiotics, 105
Bacteriostatic antibiotics, 105
Beclomethasone, 94
    dosage, 94
    structure, 87
Beta blockade, 42–43
Beta receptor, 40
    pathway, 42–43
Beta stimulation, 45
Beta sympathomimetics, 47
Bradykinin, 89
Brethine, 57–58
Bricanyl, 57–58
Bronchi: relaxation of, 45
Bronchoactive drugs, 20
Bronchoconstriction, 45
Bronchodilators
    parasympatholytic, 61–67
    sympathomimetic, 49–60
    xanthine, 61–67
Bronkosol, 56–57
Bronkotabs, 66
Buffer solutions, 33

### C

Calculation (*see* Dosages, calculation of)
Catecholamine, 49–50
    structure, 50
Cell(s)
    mast, 100, 101
    membrane function inhibition by anti-
        biotics, 104–105
    wall synthesis inhibition by antibiot-
        ics, 104
Cellular immunity, 97
Central nervous system, 35–48
    diagram of, 36
Chemical name, 2
Cholinergic, 43
Circadian rhythm, 91
CNS, 35–48
    diagram of, 36
Conversions: intersystem, 26
Corticosteroids, 83–95
    aerosol vs. oral therapy, 92–93
    anatomy of, 84–85
    control, physiology of, 88
    nucleus of, 86
    physiology of, 84–85, 88
    secretion, physiology of, 88
    structure-activity relations of, 85–86
Cortisol: diurnal variations in, 91
Cromolyn sodium, 96–103
    action site, 103

dosage, 100–101
    mechanism of, 103
Cumulation, 8
Curare, 110
Curve: log dose-response, 6
Cyclopentamine, 56
    dosage, 56
Cytophilic antibody, 100

### D

Decadron, 93
Decamethonium, 116
    dosage, 116
Decimals, 135–136
Definitions, 1
Depolarization, 111
Detergent, 78
Dexamethasone, 93
    dosage, 93
    structure, 87
Diffusion, 10
Dimethyl tubocurarine
    chloride, 114
        dosage, 114
    iodide, 115
        dosage, 115
Diurnal rhythm, 91
Dornavac, 73
Dosage
    (*See also* Dose)
    calculation of, 23–34
        mathematics of, 128–144
        from percentage-strength solutions,
            29–34
        from prepared-strength liquids, tab-
            lets and capsules, 27–29
        problems on, 142–143
        problems, conversion, 139–140
    drug potencies and, 7
    forms, 11–17
    problems, 139–140
Dose
    (*See also* Dosage)
    log dose-response curve, 6
    médian effective, 6
    median lethal, 6
    unit-dose method, 125
Drug(s)
    absorption, 9–11
    action, receptor theory of, 4–6
    bronchoactive, 20
    concepts, basic, 6–8
    cumulative amount of drug given dai-
        ly, 9
    definition of, 1
    distribution, systems of, 123–127

dosages (*see* Dosages)
efficacy of, 7
information, sources of, 3–4
interaction(s), 8–9
ionized form, 10
legislation affecting, 2
naming, 2–3
non-ionized form, 10
potency of, 7
preparation, general suggestions for, 125–126
-receptor interaction, diagrammatic representation of, 5
sources of, 3

**E**

Edema: pulmonary, and prostaglandins, 121
Efficacy of drug, 7
Elixophyllin, 65, 66
Embolism: pulmonary, and prostaglandins, 121
Ephedrine, 66
Epinephrine, 51–53
dosage, 52
racemic, 53
dosage, 53
structural formula, 51
Equivalents: approximate, 26
Ethanol, 79–80
Ethyl alcohol, 79–80

**F**

Filtration, 10
Flaxedil, 115
Fractions, 132–135
Fungal lesions: cavitary, 108

**G**

Gallamine triethiodide, 115
dosage, 115
Generic name, 3
Glucocorticoids
alternate-day therapy, 91–92
anti-inflammatory effects of, 89–90
attachments of, 86
definition, 85
diurnal rhythms and, 91–92
immunosuppression and, 90
pharmacology of, 89–93
physiologic effects of, 91
Glyceryl guaiacolate, 66
GMP, cyclic, 46

control and release, pathways of, 102
Guaifenesin, 66

**H**

Histamine release, 90
Hormone: definition, 84
Humidifiers, 14, 70–71
dosage, 70
Humoral immunity, 97
Hyperventilation: and prostaglandins, 121
Hypothalamic-pituitary-adrenal axis, 89

**I**

Idiosyncrasy, 8
IgA: secretory, 98
Immunity
cellular, 97
glucocorticoids and, 90
humoral, 97
Immunoglobulin A: secretory, 98
Immunosuppression: and glucocorticoids, 90
Index: therapeutic, 7
Inhalation route, 13–16
Inhalers, 15, 16
steam, 14
Intal, 100–103
Intersystem conversions, 26
Ipratropium bromide, 63–64
Isoetharine, 56–57
dosage, 56
structural formula, 51
Isoproterenol, 54–56
dosage, 54, 56
structural formula, 51
Isotonic solutions, 33
Isuprel, 54

**K**

Kallikrein, 89

**L**

Laplace's law, 77, 79
Law: Laplace's, 77, 79
Legislation affecting drugs, 2
Log dose-response curve, 6
Lung
edema, and prostaglandins, 121
embolism, and prostaglandins, 121
infections, gram-negative, 108
mucociliary mechanism in, 69
Lysosome rupture, 89–90

**M**

Mast cells, 100, 101
Mathematics: of dosage calculation, 128–144
Mechanical stimulation: and prostaglandins, 120–121
Mecostrin, 114
Median
  effective dose, 6
  lethal dose, 6
Medication teaching card, 20
Metaprel, 57
Metaproterenol, 52, 57
  contraindications, 57
  dosage, 57
Metric system, 23–24
Metubine, 115
Micronefrin, 53
Mineralocorticoids, 85
Mistometer aerosols, 15–16
  problems with, 59–60
Mucolytics, 68–76
  clinical use of, 74–75
Mucomyst, 71–73
Mucomyst-10, 71–73
Mucous membrane: and topical route, 16
Mucus
  nature of, 68–70
  physiology of, 68–70
  viscosity of, 69
Muscarinic effect, 43–44
Muscle relaxants, 110–116
Myoneural junction, 112
  physiology of, 111

**N**

Naming drugs, 2–3
Nebulizers, 14–15
  hand-powered, 15
Nervous system
  autonomic, 37–47
    parasympathetic branch, 37–39
    sympathetic branch, 39–43
    terminology of drugs affecting, 43–44
  central, 35–48
    diagram of, 36
  organization of, 35
  peripheral, 35–48
    diagram of, 36
Neurohormones, 38
Neuromuscular blockers, 110–116
  depolarizing, 113–114, 115–116
  nondepolarizing, 111–113, 114–115
Neurotransmitters, 38, 112

parasympathetic, 37–39
Nicotinic effect, 44
Norepinephrine, 41
  structural formula, 51
Nucleic acid synthesis: inhibition by antibiotics, 105

**O**

Official name, 2
Open-cup method, 124
Oral route, 12
Orciprenaline, 57

**P**

Pancreatic dornase, 73
  dosage, 73
Pancuronium, 115
  dosage, 115
Parasympathetic
  effects, 38
  neurotransmitters, 37–39
  stimulation, 45
Parasympatholytic(s), 39, 47
  agents, 62–64
  bronchodilators, 61–67
  definition, 43
Parasympathomimetic(s), 39
  definition, 43
Parenteral route, 12–13
Passive transfer, 10–11
Pavulon, 115
Percentage, 137–139
  means, 29
  preparations, types of, 30
  problems, solving of, 31
pH: and acetylcysteine, 72
Pharmacology
  definition of, 1
  principles of, general, 1–22
Phenobarbital, 66
Phenylephrine, 56–57
  dosage, 56
Pituitary-adrenal-hypothalamic axis, 89
Potency of drug, 7
Potentiation, 8
Prescriptions, 17–19
  abbreviations used in, 19
  parts of, 18
Prostaglandins, 117–122
  action mode, 119–120
  AMP and, cyclic, 120
  classification by major group, 118
  clinical aspects of, 120–122
  description of, 117–119
  pharmacologic effects, 119

structural aspects of, 118
terminology of, 118
Protein synthesis: inhibition by antibiotics, 105
Pulmonary (*see* Lung)

### Q

Quelicin, 115–116

### R

Ratios, 136–137
Receptor(s)
  alpha, 40
  beta, 40
    pathway of, 42–43
  theory, of drug action, 4–6
Registration number, 18
Roman numerals, 131–132
Routes of administration, 11–17
  inhalation, 13–16
  oral, 12
  parenteral, 12–13
  topical, 16–17

### S

Salbutamol, 53, 58
  dosage, 58
Separate-syringe method, 123–124
Single-syringe method, 124
Skeletal muscle relaxants, 110–116
Skin
  application, 16–17
  layers differentiating types of injection given, 13
Sodium
  bicarbonate, 73–74
    dosage, 74
  ethasulfate, 81
Solutions
  buffer, 33
  definition, 29, 33
  isotonic, 33
  mixing of, 31
  problems on, 140–142
    solving, 31–33
  by ratio, 30–31
  strength of, 29, 33
Sources: of drugs, 3
Specialized transport, 11
Sputum, 69
Steam inhaler, 14
Steroid, 85
Structure-activity relationship, 4
Succinylcholine, 115–116

dosage, 115
  sensitivity to, 113–114
Surface-active agents, 77–82
  clinical consideration of, 81–82
Surface tension, 77–78, 79
Sympathetic effects, 39
Sympatholytic(s), 43
  alpha, 47
Sympathomimetic(s), 43
  activity of, spectrum of, 41
  beta, 47
  bronchodilators, 49–60
Syncurine, 116
Synergism, 8
Systems: of drug distribution, 123–127

### T

Tachyphylaxis, 9
Terbutaline, 52, 57–58
  dosage, 58
Tergemist, 81
Theophylline
  in Bronkotabs, 66
  capsules, 65
    dosage, 65
  elixir, 66
    dosage, 66
  ethylenediamine, 65
    dosage, 65
  with guaifenesin, 66
Therapeutic index, 7
Tolerance, 9
Topical route, 16–17
Trade name, 3
Transport: specialized, 11
Triamcinolone, 94–95
Tubocurarine chloride, 114
*d*-Tubocurarine, 114
  dosage, 114
Tyloxapol, 80
  dosage, 80

### U

Unit-dose method, 125

### V

Vanceril, 94
Vaponefrin, 53
Vaporizer, 14

### X

Xanthine
  agents, 64–66
  bronchodilators, 61–67